Depression Conceptuali

Depression Conceptualization and Treatment

Christos Charis • Georgia Panayiotou
Editors

Depression Conceptualization and Treatment

Dialogues from Psychodynamic
and Cognitive Behavioral Perspectives

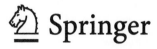 Springer

Editors
Christos Charis
Private Practice
Dillenburg, Germany

Georgia Panayiotou
Department of Psychology and Center
of Applied Neuroscience
University of Cyprus
Nicosia, Cyprus

ISBN 978-3-030-68934-6   ISBN 978-3-030-68932-2   (eBook)
https://doi.org/10.1007/978-3-030-68932-2

This Springer imprint is published by the registered company Springer Nature Switzerland AG
The registered company address is: Gewerbestrasse 11, 6330 Cham, Switzerland

General Introduction

Depression, a highly common clinical disorder, is an important and clinically relevant topic for both clinical researchers and practitioners to address, because of its prevalence, impact on the individual and society, association with other mental and physical health problems, and the social contexts in which it develops. Depression ranks in Germany and Central Europe as the third among the leading mental disorders and it is a leading cause of disability worldwide. It is estimated that 8.3% of the German population is depressed within a year (11.2% women, 5.5% men). These statistics mean that four million people per year are depressed in Germany alone (1 year prevalence). According to the WHO, over 300 million people worldwide experience depression and in the USA the financial burden of this disorder, due to disability, work absenteeism, medical and other costs reaches over 210 billion dollars annually. Depression is also becoming more frequent over time and has a high risk of recidivism—particularly since its most common form, Major Depressive Disorder (DSM-5; ICD10), tends to occur in episodes. For example, 20–40% of people become depressed again within 2 years after their first depressive episode, meaning that a major aim of any therapeutic intervention should be to prevent future relapses. Depression also shows very high comorbidities with other mental and physical health conditions. Its overlap with anxiety pathology is so high that clinicians are concerned whether the two disorder categories are indeed distinct or if they show substantial etiological overlap. Depression is also associated with heart disease and even cancer, making it a risk factor for mortality and morbidity that needs to be identified early and addressed effectively. In addition to major depressive disorder, the often severe bipolar disorder and the chronic form of depression referred to as dysthymia are additional mood disorders that among them require careful differential diagnosis. They also evoke questions regarding their common or distinct etiological mechanisms.

In order to gain a better understanding of depression as a clinical disorder, one needs to look at it as a multifaceted phenomenon. Depression is a neurobehavioral condition, and one has to be up to date and have a solid understanding of its biological substrate, at a genetic, neuronal, hormonal, and pharmacological level. Depression is also a socio-demographic phenomenon, and one needs to examine its epidemiology that might contain significant cues toward its clearer understanding. It is more prevalent, for example, in certain regions, climates, age groups, and genders (much more prevalent in women, with age of appearance in young adulthood but also presents as a significant problem for youth and the elderly), is associated with stereotypes and stigma, and can be the aftermath of crises, trauma, and loss.

The etiology of depression remains under scrutiny, though recently much more knowledge is emerging from contemporary neuroimaging, genotyping, and data science methods. Different neural and behavioral systems may be involved in contributing to the significant heterogeneity within the disorder. Social roles, stressors, attachment patterns, family support and social networks, and individual (e.g., gender linked) vulnerabilities may contribute significantly toward increasing risk for developing depression. Different therapeutic approaches, like those stemming from the psychoanalytic/psychodynamic perspectives and those stemming from the cognitive/behavioral (second and third wave) traditions, focus on the components of etiology considered most dominant. As science progresses with clearer evidence regarding the important etiological factors and their interactions, these different perspectives, each with its own contribution, may need to take new developments into consideration, adapt and even begin to converge.

These different aspects of the topic of depression, which are central to the scientific aims of clinical scientists, but also permeate the way clinicians approach assessment, diagnosis, case formulation, and treatment, become the focus of the present volume. Following a conference held at the University of Cyprus, in Nicosia, Cyprus, in October 2019, which included presentations by internationally renowned experts in the field on these various aspects of depression, the idea of extending the topics presented and discussed at the meeting into more elaborate and substantive chapters and synthesizing them into an edited volume was generated. The aim was to fill a substantive gap, with a volume that would be beneficial to a wider, interdisciplinary audience of clinicians, trainees, and researchers who examine the different aspects of depression.

In this edited volume, with contributions from prominent experts in the field, we propose to discuss the subject of conceptualizing and treating depression and related conditions (e.g., suicide, bipolar disorder) from different theoretical perspectives and after taking into consideration current research into the etiology and maintenance of this condition. Chapters on theoretical perspectives of treatment cover a wide range of approaches, which could be broadly clustered under behavioral and psychodynamic points of view. Perspectives discussed in this volume are psychodynamic therapy, second wave CBT, acceptance and commitment therapy, and mentalization therapy. Special topics with great relevance to treatment include treatment in different levels of care (e.g., partial hospital setting, prevention of suicide, working with cancer patients). The book provides a unique combination of current empirical findings on the etiology of depression and suicide, treatment considerations and practical recommendations, treatment in different settings, and combination of different theoretical perspectives that can enrich a therapists' repertoire of tools for understanding and approaching depression. The book describes various theoretical approaches without adhering to any one but with an effort to highlight common underlying themes like issues of loss, self-esteem, guilt, grief, and emotion regulation as these permeate the various perspectives. In this way the book presents a combination of science and practice and of various views that constitute an excellent resource for researchers, clinicians, and students of mental health professions. In a final chapter the two editors, Drs. Christos Charis and Georgia Panayiotou, make an effort to impartially integrate information from various perspectives, highlighting the utility of each approach to address specific vulnerability and etiological factors discussed in the book. In this regard, the volume stresses the idea of the need for continuous and open dialogue between perspectives, theories, levels of investigation, research areas, practitioner needs, and scientific views to help make progress in treatment and address this complex and multifaceted phenomenon in the service of patients, their carers, and societies in general.

Contents

Chapter 1
Neurodevelopmental Aspects of Suicide

Andreas Chatzittofis

Contents

Suicide is the fatal result of a self-injurious act of which there is some evidence of the intent to die. A suicide attempt is the behavior that is considered potentially self-injurious with at least some intent to die (Turecki & Brent, 2016).

Both suicide and suicide attempts are currently a major health problem. According to the World Health Organization (WHO), there are more than 800,000 suicide victims every year, making suicide the second leading cause of death in young people aged 15–29 (WHO, 2019). Approximately, there is an annual global age-standardized suicide rate of 10.5 per 100,000 population. There are differences between different countries and cultures. There are more young adults and elderly women suicide victims in low-income countries than in high-income countries. However, middle-aged men have much higher suicide rates in high-income countries than in low-income countries (WHO, 2019). Regarding gender, men are approximately four times more likely to die from suicide compared to women although there is a variation between different areas in the world. On the contrary, women are more likely to make a suicide attempt compared to men. This discrepancy is thought to be related to the different suicide methods used by men and women. Men tend to use more violent methods such as hanging and firearms

A. Chatzittofis (✉)
School of Medicine, University of Cyprus, Nicosia, Cyprus
e-mail: chatzittofis.andreas@ucy.ac.cy

© Springer Nature Switzerland AG 2021
C. Charis, G. Panayiotou (eds.), *Depression Conceptualization and Treatment*,
https://doi.org/10.1007/978-3-030-68932-2_1

1

compared to women who use less lethal methods such as overdosing medication. But also differences in culture, rates of mental illness, as well as access and utilization of health care may impact these sex differences (Nock et al., 2008).

Suicidal behavior is related to psychopathology, especially mood disorders, addiction, psychosis, and personality disorders. Suicide attempts are a larger public health issue, with at least 10–20 times the number of suicides. A history of a suicide attempt is the most important risk factor for a subsequent completed suicide. Consequently, suicide became a priority in the WHO Mental Health Action Plan 2013–2020 aiming at a 10% decrease in the rate of suicide by 2020. Another close related issue is the nonfatal nonsuicidal self-injurious (NSSI) behavior, meaning intentional self-injurious behavior but with the absence of suicide intent. It includes cutting, burning, banging or hitting, and scratching one's own body tissue. Especially the last years, there has been an increase of the phenomenon with younger age of onset. NSSI is highly prevalent among female adolescents, with lifetime prevalence rates around 20%, and has a close relationship with suicidal behaviors (Cipriano, Cella, & Cotrufo, 2017).

1.1 Risk Factors for Suicide

Suicide is a major health problem, and thus there is an imperative need to identify both risk factors and biomarkers in order to apply preventive measures. If individuals at risk can be identified, underlying disorders can be treated, and resilience measures can be applied in order to lower the suicide risk for vulnerable individuals.

Indeed, research has identified a lot of risk factors. Some demographic risk factors are gender with males being at higher risk and age with suicide rates increasing with advanced age. Moreover, other factors such as lower socioeconomic status, migration, unemployment, and divorce also increase the risk for suicide.

Studies of psychological autopsies highlight the importance of psychopathology with more than 90% of suicide victims diagnosed with a psychiatric illness, most commonly mood disorders, especially depression, psychosis, alcohol and substance abuse, as well as borderline personality disorder. Even physical illnesses, especially painful disorders, are considered to be a risk factor. Besides diagnoses, some psychiatric symptoms and traits have been shown to be related with suicidal behavior. These are feelings of hopelessness, impulsivity, and aggression but also social isolation. Violence is also an important risk factor, and it is more obvious with high rates of suicide among prisoners and in forensic settings. Finally, the suicidal process by itself is a risk factor. Suicidal ideation, a previous suicide attempt, recurrent suicide attempts, as well as a violent suicide method are related to increase suicide risk.

Last but not least, childhood adversity is considered a very important risk factor for developing psychopathology in adulthood and more specifically for suicide (Teicher & Samson, 2013; van Heeringen & Mann, 2014).

This has been shown previously in the literature and for different types of childhood abuse including emotional and physical abuse and neglect as well sexual abuse. Thus, suicide can be considered as a disorder with childhood onset (Turecki, Ernst, Jollant, Labonte, & Mechawar, 2012).

Some of the risk factors for suicide are static such as the genetic background and family history of suicide. However, there are also dynamic factors such as social support and presence of psychopathology, for example, a depressive episode, that are susceptible to change. A typical example is the effective treatment of psychiatric disorders. But most importantly, even childhood adversity, a known risk factor, can be decreased when applying the right measures earlier in life.

1.2 Model of Suicidal Behavior

In order to understand suicide and suicidal behavior, Turecki and Brent (2016) proposed a model integrating the known risk factors involved. This model can be seen from a developmental perspective, meaning that suicide process has its origins long before the appearance of suicidal behavior and different risk factors have an impact in different points on time and not necessarily directly preceding suicidal behavior.

This stress-diathesis model for suicidal behavior has been proposed earlier by Mann (2003) and gives the possibility to illustrate the relationship between different biological systems with clinical correlates of suicidal behavior (Mann, 2003; van Heeringen & Mann, 2014). Known risk factors for suicide can be categorized into three groups (Turecki & Brent, 2016).

The first group is the distal factors, often mentioned in the patient's history. These factors contribute to the predisposition to suicidal behavior and include a family history of suicide, a childhood adversity, and the genetic background of the individual. It is already known that there is a very important interaction between the genetic background and environmental factors such as stressful life events (Caspi et al., 2003).

The second group includes developmental factors that mediate the effect of the distal factors to suicidal behavior. In this category, personality traits as well as cognitive styles are found. These include aggression, impulsivity, anxiety traits, as well as deficits in decision-making and problem-solving (Hawton & van Heeringen, 2009; Turecki, 2014; Turecki & Brent, 2016).

Finally, for the third group, we have the proximal, to the suicide event, risk factors that are mainly responsible for triggering suicidal behavior. Recent life events such as a psychosocial crisis due to the exposure to acute stress, the availability of means to commit suicide, isolation, and lack of social support may trigger the suicidal behavior (Fig. 1.1) (Turecki & Brent, 2016).

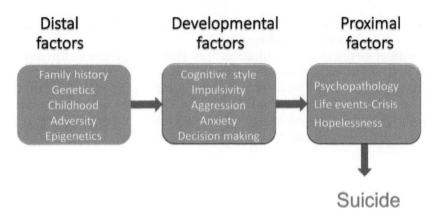

Fig. 1.1 Stress-diathesis model of suicidal behavior

1.3 Biomarkers Suicide and Childhood Adversity

Along with all the abovementioned clinical features and risk factors for suicide, different biomarkers have been identified to be related with suicidal behavior. These biomarkers are identified from structural brain imaging studies as well as genetic and biochemical studies. Focus has been on the hypothalamic-pituitary-adrenal (HPA) axis as the major stress system regulator but also neuroinflammation and neurotransmitters such as serotonin and catecholamines. Briefly, at the presence of a stressor, the corticotropin-releasing hormone (CRH) is released from the paraventricular nucleus of the hypothalamus. This subsequently triggers the secretion of adrenocorticotropic hormone (ACTH) from the pituitary gland. As a result, glucocorticoids are produced by the adrenal cortex that have the ability to regulate the secretion of ACTH and CRH through inhibitory loops to achieve homeostasis. Glucocorticoids act by binding to the glucocorticoid receptor (GR) and the mineralocorticoid receptor (MR) in different areas in the brain, including the hypothalamus and prefrontal cortex, and regulating metabolism, the immune system, as well as cognition (De Bellis & Zisk, 2014).

Here, we are going to discuss some novel biomarkers for suicide in relation to childhood adversity and more specifically HPA axis, the serotonergic system, and the oxytocin system.

1.4 HPA Axis

The most common finding in adults with history of childhood adversity is low levels of plasma cortisol (De Bellis & Zisk, 2014; Heim, Newport, Bonsall, Miller, & Nemeroff, 2001). The dexamethasone suppression test (DST) has been used to test the function of the HPA axis (Carroll, Martin, & Davies, 1968). In order to test the inhibition induced to cortisol production, a synthetic glucocorticoid, dexamethasone, is given. If the production of cortisol is not suppressed, as one would expect, then the individual is characterized as non-suppressor, indicating a dysfunction of the HPA axis. According to the review by Coryell, completed suicide is associated with higher rates of DST non-suppressors, i.e., hyperactivity of the HPA axis (Coryell, 2012; Coryell & Schlesser, 2001; Jokinen et al., 2007; Jokinen, Nordstrom, & Nordstrom, 2009). On the other hand, Pfennig et al. (2005) reported a lower adrenocorticotropin and cortisol response in the combined Dex/CRH test, especially in depressed patients with suicidal behavior. The HPA dysfunction has also been shown with increased CRH in the cerebrospinal fluid of suicide victims and with reduced sites in the frontal cortex for the binding of CRH in suicide victims (Arato, Banki, Bissette, & Nemeroff, 1989; Nemeroff, Owens, Bissette, Andorn, & Stanley, 1988).

The mechanism that increases the risk for psychopathology in adult life is suggested to be via the long-standing effects and alternation of the neurobiological systems that occur due to the exposure to childhood adversity (De Bellis & Zisk, 2014; Lupien, McEwen, Gunnar, & Heim, 2009; Turecki, 2014; Turecki et al., 2012; van Heeringen & Mann, 2014). Thus, homeostasis of the neurobiological systems is dysregulated with functional consequences in adult life. In fact, not only 12 different mechanisms are proposed in how childhood adversity affects the HPA axis but also other neurobiological systems that are involved such as the serotonin system and the oxytocin system (De Bellis & Zisk, 2014).

It is suggested that early-life trauma sensitizes the HPA axis resulting in higher cortisol levels in response to stress later in life. In the same line, Heim et al. showed increased cortisol and adrenocorticotropin hormone (ACTH) responses at the dexamethasone/corticotropin-releasing factor (CRF) test in depressed men with a history of childhood abuse compared to healthy controls and depressed men without a history of childhood abuse (Heim, Mletzko, Purselle, Musselman, & Nemeroff, 2008; Heim, Newport, Mletzko, Miller, & Nemeroff, 2008).

It is important to mention that individual differences, the gender, the timing of the trauma, duration, and severity as well as genetic, epigenetic, and social factors are important in the development of the effects of the trauma on the biological systems and psychopathology (De Bellis & Zisk, 2014).

There are a lot of examples of gene-environment interaction regarding childhood adversity. Childhood adversity and especially sexual abuse and emotional neglect were shown to interact with the CRH receptor gene on decision-making in suicide attempters (Guillaume et al., 2013). Moreover, childhood adversity showed an interaction with a gene related to stress by moderating the activation of the glucocorticoid receptor (FKBP5) in the prediction of risk for suicide attempt (A. Roy, Gorodetsky, Yuan, Goldman, & Enoch, 2010).

1.5   Serotonin System

The other most profound/replicated neurobiological correlate of suicidal behavior has been with the hypofunction of the serotonin system, indicated by lower levels of 5-hydroxyindoleacetic acid (5-HIAA), the main metabolite of serotonin, in the cerebrospinal fluid (Asberg, Traskman, & Thoren, 1976; Chatzittofis et al., 2013; Mann & Currier, 2007; Oquendo et al., 2014; van Heeringen & Mann, 2014). The role of serotonin in depression is also established. Besides serotonin's effect on depression, the impact of this hypofunction of the serotonergic system on behavior is suggested as traits like aggression and impulsivity with impairment in inhibition that contributes to the vulnerability to committing suicide (Rosell & Siever, 2015; Turecki, 2014). The question of trait or state of the low 5-HIAA in suicide has been ongoing (Asberg, Nordstrom, & Traskman-Bendz, 1986). It is important to point out that the different biological systems are closely related to each other, and thus a number of different biomarkers would be more suitable to identify a "biosignature for suicide" and therefore the individuals who are at risk (Guintivano et al., 2014; Kaminsky et al., 2015; Niculescu et al., 2015; Oquendo et al., 2014).

Regarding gene polymorphisms of the serotonergic system, it has been reported that gene variation can moderate the relationship between childhood trauma, depression, and suicidal behavior (Brodsky, 2016). A number of studies show that childhood adversity has been related to low-expressing 5-HTTLPR genotypes and increased risk for suicide attempts in different populations such as bipolar, substance dependence, and adult inpatients. However, as findings are inconsistent, there is a need for further research regarding the relationship between childhood adversity and serotonin genetic variations that can lead to suicidal behavior.

1.6   Oxytocin

Oxytocin is a neuropeptide implicated in social interaction and behaviors such as affiliation, trust, and aggression and has an important role in early attachment (Heinrichs, von Dawans, & Domes, 2009; Insel, 2010; Neumann, 2009; Olff, 2012). In the central nervous system, oxytocin has its effects in the hypothalamus, cortex, brainstem, olfactory areas, and amygdala and implicated in depression, anxiety, autism, fear, and resilience to stress (Heinrichs et al., 2009; Pierrehumbert et al., 2010; Veening, de Jong, & Barendregt, 2010). Oxytocin is also important in stress regulation and interacts with the HPA axis in an inhibitory manner (Neumann, Krömer, Toschi, & Ebner, 2000; Petersson, Hulting, & Uvnas-Moberg, 1999; Windle et al., 2004; Windle, Shanks, Lightman, & Ingram, 1997).

As oxytocin is involved in the stress response and has major effects on social behavior, it is reasonable to assume that it has also a role in suicidal behavior. Indeed, there is some evidence that oxytocin is involved in suicide. A study reported that CSF oxytocin was inversely correlated with life history of aggression, a known risk factor for suicide (Lee, Ferris, Van de Kar, & Coccaro, 2009). Interestingly, through an exploratory analysis, lower levels of CSF oxytocin were found in suicide attempters compared to patients with no history of suicidal behavior (Lee et al., 2009).

The oxytocin system is also closely related to early adversity-related psychopathology (De Bellis & Zisk, 2014). Lower CSF oxytocin concentrations were reported in women with a history of childhood abuse compared with women without childhood abuse (Heim et al., 2009). Similarly, in healthy men, plasma oxytocin levels were negatively associated with early-life adverse experiences (Opacka-Juffry & Mohiyeddini, 2012), and likewise in another study, a negative correlation between plasma oxytocin levels and childhood trauma when investigating women with borderline personality disorder was reported (Bertsch, Schmidinger, Neumann, & Herpertz, 2013). Findings remain contradictory with another study reporting that abused women had higher baseline oxytocin levels and premature suppression of oxytocin in a study using the Trier Social Stress Test (Pierrehumbert et al., 2010). In the same line, high levels of oxytocin secretion were reported only in girls with a history of childhood abuse that underwent the Trier Social Stress Test, while there was no difference in boys (Seltzer, Ziegler, Connolly, Prososki, & Pollak, 2014). Although there are contradicting results, there is consensus regarding the possible effect of both genetic and epigenetic factors on the oxytocin system (De Bellis & Zisk, 2014; Herpertz & Bertsch, 2015; Seltzer et al., 2014). Genetic factors such as the oxytocin transporter rs2254298 polymorphism were reported to interact with early adversity and predict anxiety and depressive symptoms (Thompson, Parker, Hallmayer, Waugh, & Gotlib, 2011). Cicchetti et al. reported a three-way interaction between maltreatment, gender, and genetic variants of the OXTR genotype in predicting borderline symptomatology (Cicchetti, Rogosch, Hecht, Crick, & Hetzel, 2014). Bradley et al. reported an interaction between the oxytocin receptor gene polymorphism OXTR rs53576 and a positive family environment in predicting resilient coping and positive affect (Bradley, Davis, Wingo, Mercer, & Ressler, 2013). Finally, a model was proposed for the pathophysiology of borderline personality disorder in which oxytocin has a central role affecting among others the social approach behavior and affect regulation (Herpertz & Bertsch, 2015).

In addition, there are also reports on oxytocin and suicide specifically. Lower CSF oxytocin levels were also reported in suicide attempters with high suicide intent compared to suicide attempters with low suicide attempt (Jokinen et al., 2012). The lower oxytocin in the suicide attempters might reflect a deficit in prosocial behavior leading to an impaired social support network that increases the risk for suicidal behavior. Additionally, it might be related to suicide through stress regulation and cognitive deficits such as in decision-making. Oxytocin is implicated in stress regulation, regulates stress in relation to social interaction, and has an inhibitory effect on the HPA axis (Heinrichs, Baumgartner, Kirschbaum, & Ehlert, 2003; Neumann, 2009). Additionally, suicide attempters have "cognitive rigidity" (Neuringer, 1964) as well as deficits in decision-making when making choices under uncertainty (Jollant et al., 2010; Turecki & Brent, 2016). A number of genes associated with the oxytocin system and affiliative behavior were also associated with autism spectrum disorders (Yrigollen et al., 2008), and infusions of oxytocin can reduce repetitive behavior in adults with autistic traits and Asperger syndrome (Hollander et al., 2003). Regarding childhood adversity, significantly lower oxytocin plasma levels were reported in revictimized suicide attempters compared to nonrevictimized suicide attempters (Chatzittofis, Nordstrom, Uvnas-Moberg, Asberg, & Jokinen, 2014). Being a victim of violence in childhood is associated with higher risk for revictimization in adult life (Widom, Czaja, & Dutton, 2008).

1.7   Epigenetics, Childhood Adversity, and Suicide

Epigenetic studies reveal the impact of childhood adversity on suicidal behavior. Epigenetics may be mediating the effects of early-life adversity on behavior. This can be seen by alternations of DNA methylation in gene regulatory regions which, in turn, has been associated with changes in gene expression and behavioral modifications. Regarding epigenetic mechanisms, a study more than a decade ago reported increased methylation in a neuron-specific glucocorticoid receptor (NR3C1) promoter and lower levels of hippocampal glucocorticoid receptor expression in suicide victims with a history of childhood abuse compared to suicide victims without a history of child abuse (McGowan et al., 2009). Subsequently, DNA methylation alterations at the hippocampal glucocorticoid receptor promoter were reported in abused suicide victims, supporting that childhood adversity induces long-lasting effects (Labonte et al., 2012).

Moreover, depressed patients and more specifically patients with severe suicidal ideation had significantly hypermethylated FK506-binding protein 5 (FKBP5), corticotropin releasing hormone binding protein (CRHBP), and glucocorticoid receptor gene (NR3C1) promoters (B. Roy, Shelton, & Dwivedi, 2017).

In another study, suicide attempters with high-risk phenotype had lower levels of methylation in the promoter region of the CRH gene and more specifically, at two methylation loci, i.e., cg19035496 and cg23409074, compared to suicide attempters exposed to less serious suicide attempts (Jokinen et al., 2018). Even in a genome-wide methylation study in the brains of suicide completers, the authors reported that 366 promoters were differentially methylated in suicide completers compared to controls. These methylation differences were inversely correlated with gene expression, and these genes were involved in cognitive processes (Labonté et al., 2013). This was verified by a meta-analysis of DNA methylation data of brains of suicide completers, suggesting that it is associated with suicide (Policicchio et al., 2020).

Thus, early-life adversity through effects on the epigenetic regulation of HPA axis affects the development of stable emotional, behavioral, and cognitive phenotypes and increases the risk of suicide (Turecki, Ota, Belangero, Jackowski, & Kaufman, 2014).

1.8   Transgenerational Transmission

We have discussed the role of childhood trauma on psychopathology and more specifically on suicidal behavior. But when does the vulnerability for suicide start? Is it in childhood or is it possible that childhood adversity of the parents has an impact on the offspring? Indeed, there are some studies that report that epigenetics changes of the parents due to maltreatment pass on to the offspring; thus, there is a transgenerational transmission. In a study on the Holocaust, the authors studied cytosine methylation within the gene encoding for FK506 binding protein 5 (FKBP5) in Holocaust survivors and their adult offspring. This was compared with control parents and their offspring, respectively. They reported that methylation levels for exposed parents and their offspring were significantly correlated and that there is a site specificity to environmental influences, with some sites associated with the offspring's own childhood trauma, and others with parental trauma (Yehuda et al., 2016). Moreover, intergenerational effects of the Holocaust have been found regarding cortisol levels (Dashorst, Mooren, Kleber, de Jong, & Huntjens, 2019). Likewise, when studying the Tutsi genocide and posttraumatic stress disorder, similar epigenetic modifications of the glucocorticoid receptor (GR) gene (NR3C1) were found in the mothers and their offspring (Perroud et al., 2014). However, these results are preliminary, and further research is needed to elucidate the possible mechanisms of transgenerational transmission.

1.9   Prevention and Treatment

Prevention is the most important when dealing a complex phenomenon with detrimental consequences as suicide. Unfortunately, we have not yet established a reliable prediction model for suicide.

The World Health Organization recommends specific actions that can have an effect in reducing suicide rates when applied at a population level. The key to effective suicide prevention is a comprehensive multisector approach through a national suicide prevention strategy. First, it is important to minimize access to the means of suicide, most specifically pesticides that are highly toxic. This measure is already applied in many countries. Using firearms is another way people attempt suicide. Thus, firearm control is very important to counteract violence as well as suicide. Second is developing effective coping skills to life's pressures in young people. This aims to reduce the impact of different adverse events on mental health that might trigger suicide attempts. Third, WHO recommends preventive measures targeting specific populations at risk. Early identification and management of people at risk like suicide attempters is of high importance. Effective treatment with follow-up that would minimize suicide risk should be applied. The same principles should be used in all psychiatric disorders. As the majority of suicide victims have an identified psychiatric disorder, psychiatric services should be vigilant for any signs of increased suicide risk. Finally, interaction with the media in order to achieve responsible reporting of suicide is also necessary. This aims eliminating any sensationalist articles by training and awareness for media professionals and promoting positive reporting such as resilience stories and eliminating stigma. It is important that interventions are school and community based to increase their effect. When evaluating suicide from a developmental aspect, it becomes obvious that some interventions are critical and can have a delayed effect. Such as an example is the effort to decrease and eliminate childhood adversity, therefore minimizing vulnerability to adult psychopathology and to suicidal behavior.

1.10 Conclusions

Suicide and suicidal behavior is a complex phenomenon with high impact on society. The stress-diathesis model with distal, mediator, and proximal risk factors is applied to understand suicidal behavior. This model is also integrated with biological systems and biomarkers such as HPA axis and serotonin and oxytocin systems. Childhood adversity has been identified as a major risk factor for suicide, and it supported to be mediated through alternations of biological systems such as the HPA axis and the oxytocin system. These are long-lasting alternations mediated via epigenetic mechanisms. Although a lot of promising biomarkers have been identified, it is still very difficult to make predictions. It is important to understand the process of suicidal behavior in order to apply both preventive and therapeutic measures. And preventive measures can be applied especially in targeting vulnerable populations and policies such as access to firearms and pesticides. Childhood adversity is an ideal target for prevention and should be included as a priority when discussing measures against suicide.

1.11 Case

Situation A young 24-year-old woman is seeking medical care at the emergency department at midnight. She is accompanied by a friend and informs the doctor that she took about 20 tablets of alprazolam of 1 mg 1 h prior to her arrival at the emergency department. What preceded the incidence was a fight with her boyfriend who wanted to end the relationship. After being treated, the emergency department refers the patient to the on-call psychiatrist for an assessment. She now wants to go home and forget what happened.

Background The patient was raised in an orphanage from the age of 2 followed by a foster family between ages 10 and 17. She finished high school but did not continue with higher education but has been working in sales the last years. The patient is currently unemployed (lost her job 1 month ago) and lives with her parents and occasionally with her boyfriend. She had multiple unstable relationships through the years, the longer relationship was 4 months, and she has been in her current relationship for the last 3 months.

Psychiatric History Her first contact with mental health services was in her early teens due to disruptive behavior and oppositional disorder. In her late teens, she developed anorexia nervosa and now has more bulimic symptoms. Through the years, she also presented periodic alcohol abuse. The patient is currently diagnosed with borderline personality disorder and is treated with antidepressants, antipsychotics, and benzodiazepines (alprazolam). This is her fifth suicide attempt. The first was when she was 17 years old and the last one 6 months ago. All suicide attempts were through medication overdose.

Assessment and Discussion In this case, it is obvious that this is a chronic situation with suicidal behavior with exacerbations. We can identify a lot of risk factors such as childhood adversity, impulsivity, aggression, substance abuse, as well as psychopathology. Finally, we have the crisis that triggers the suicidal behavior. She has also access to the means to commit suicide (medication). A targeted treatment plan would focus on treating underlying psychopathology with psychotherapy, minimizing access to means (stopping unnecessary medication and strict prescription of small amounts of medication), increasing coping skills to life stressors, and establishing a supportive social network to the patient.

References

Arato, M., Banki, C. M., Bissette, G., & Nemeroff, C. B. (1989). Elevated CSF CRF in suicide victims. *Biological Psychiatry, 25*(3), 355–359. 0006-3223(89)90183-2 [pii].

Asberg, M., Nordstrom, P., & Traskman-Bendz, L. (1986). Cerebrospinal fluid studies in suicide. An overview. *Annals of the New York Academy of Sciences, 487,* 243–255.

Asberg, M., Traskman, L., & Thoren, P. (1976). 5-HIAA in the cerebrospinal fluid. A biochemical suicide predictor? *Archives of General Psychiatry, 33*(10), 1193–1197.

Bertsch, K., Schmidinger, I., Neumann, I. D., & Herpertz, S. C. (2013). Reduced plasma oxytocin levels in female patients with borderline personality disorder. *Hormones and Behavior, 63*(3), 424–429.

Bradley, B., Davis, T. A., Wingo, A. P., Mercer, K. B., & Ressler, K. J. (2013). Family environment and adult resilience: Contributions of positive parenting and the oxytocin receptor gene. *European Journal of Psychotraumatology, 4.*

Brodsky, B. S. (2016). Early childhood environment and genetic interactions: The diathesis for suicidal behavior. *Current Psychiatry Reports, 18*(9), 86.

Carroll, B. J., Martin, F. I., & Davies, B. (1968). Resistance to suppression by dexamethasone of plasma 11-O.H.C.S. levels in severe depressive illness. *British Medical Journal, 3*(5613), 285–287.

Caspi, A., Sugden, K., Moffitt, T. E., Taylor, A., Craig, I. W., Harrington, H., ... Poulton, R. (2003). Influence of life stress on depression: Moderation by a polymorphism in the 5-HTT gene. *Science, 301*(5631), 386–389.

Chatzittofis, A., Nordstrom, P., Hellstrom, C., Arver, S., Asberg, M., & Jokinen, J. (2013). CSF 5-HIAA, cortisol and DHEAS levels in suicide attempters. *European Neuropsychopharmacology, 23*(10), 1280–1287. https://doi.org/10.1016/j.euroneuro.2013.02.002

Chatzittofis, A., Nordstrom, P., Uvnas-Moberg, K., Asberg, M., & Jokinen, J. (2014). CSF and plasma oxytocin levels in suicide attempters, the role of childhood trauma and revictimization. *Neuroendocrinology Letters, 35*(3), 213–217.

Cicchetti, D., Rogosch, F. A., Hecht, K. F., Crick, N. R., & Hetzel, S. (2014). Moderation of maltreatment effects on childhood borderline personality symptoms by gender and oxytocin receptor and FK506 binding protein 5 genes. *Developmental Psychopathology, 26*(3), 831–849.

Cipriano, A., Cella, S., & Cotrufo, P. (2017). Nonsuicidal self-injury: A systematic review. *Frontiers in Psychology, 8*, 1946. https://doi.org/10.3389/fpsyg.2017.01946

Coryell, W. (2012). Do serum cholesterol values and DST results comprise independent risk factors for suicide? In *The neurobiological basis of suicide*. Boca Raton, FL: CRC Press/Taylor & Francis. NBK107215.

Coryell, W., & Schlesser, M. (2001). The dexamethasone suppression test and suicide prediction. *American Journal of Psychiatry, 158*(5), 748–753.

Dashorst, P., Mooren, T. M., Kleber, R. J., de Jong, P. J., & Huntjens, R. J. C. (2019). Intergenerational consequences of the Holocaust on offspring mental health: A systematic review of associated factors and mechanisms. *European Jouranl of Psychotraumatology, 10*(1), 1654065. https://doi.org/10.1080/20008198.2019.1654065

De Bellis, M. D., & Zisk, A. (2014). The biological effects of childhood trauma. *Child and Adolescent Psychiatric Clinics, 23*(2), 185–222.

Guillaume, S., Perroud, N., Jollant, F., Jaussent, I., Olie, E., Malafosse, A., & Courtet, P. (2013). HPA axis genes may modulate the effect of childhood adversities on decision-making in suicide attempters. *Journal of Psychiatry Research, 47*(2), 259–265.

Guintivano, J., Brown, T., Newcomer, A., Jones, M., Cox, O., Maher, B. S., … Kaminsky, Z. A. (2014). Identification and replication of a combined epigenetic and genetic biomarker predicting suicide and suicidal behaviors. *American Journal of Psychiatry, 171*(12), 1287–1296.

Hawton, K., & van Heeringen, K. (2009). Suicide. *Lancet, 373*(9672), 1372–1381.

Heim, C., Mletzko, T., Purselle, D., Musselman, D. L., & Nemeroff, C. B. (2008). The dexamethasone/corticotropin-releasing factor test in men with major depression: Role of childhood trauma. *Biological Psychiatry, 63*(4), 398–405.

Heim, C., Newport, D. J., Bonsall, R., Miller, A. H., & Nemeroff, C. B. (2001). Altered pituitary-adrenal axis responses to provocative challenge tests in adult survivors of childhood abuse. *American Journal of Psychiatry, 158*(4), 575–581.

Heim, C., Newport, D. J., Mletzko, T., Miller, A. H., & Nemeroff, C. B. (2008). The link between childhood trauma and depression: Insights from HPA axis studies in humans. *Psychoneuroendocrinology, 33*(6), 693–710.

Heim, C., Young, L. J., Newport, D. J., Mletzko, T., Miller, A. H., & Nemeroff, C. B. (2009). Lower CSF oxytocin concentrations in women with a history of childhood abuse. *Molecular Psychiatry, 14*(10), 954–958.

Heinrichs, M., Baumgartner, T., Kirschbaum, C., & Ehlert, U. (2003). Social support and oxytocin interact to suppress cortisol and subjective responses to psychosocial stress. *Biological Psychiatry, 54*(12), 1389–1398.

Heinrichs, M., von Dawans, B., & Domes, G. (2009). Oxytocin, vasopressin, and human social behavior. *Frontiers in Neuroendocrinology, 30*(4), 548–557.

Herpertz, S. C., & Bertsch, K. (2015). A new perspective on the pathophysiology of borderline personality disorder: A model of the role of oxytocin. *American Journal of Psychiatry, 172*(9), 840–851.

Hollander, E., Novotny, S., Hanratty, M., Yaffe, R., DeCaria, C. M., Aronowitz, B. R., & Mosovich, S. (2003). Oxytocin infusion reduces repetitive behaviors in adults with autistic and Asperger's disorders. *Neuropsychopharmacology, 28*(1), 193–198.

Insel, T. R. (2010). The challenge of translation in social neuroscience: A review of oxytocin, vasopressin, and affiliative behavior. *Neuron, 65*(6), 768–779.

Jokinen, J., Boström, A. E., Dadfar, A., Ciuculete, D. M., Chatzittofis, A., Åsberg, M., & Schiöth, H. B. (2018). Epigenetic changes in the CRH gene are related to severity of suicide attempt and a general psychiatric risk score in adolescents. *eBioMedicine, 27*, 123–133.

Jokinen, J., Carlborg, A., Martensson, B., Forslund, K., Nordstrom, A. L., & Nordstrom, P. (2007). DST non-suppression predicts suicide after attempted suicide. *Psychiatry Research, 150*(3), 297–303.

Jokinen, J., Chatzittofis, A., Hellström, C., Nordström, P., Uvnäs-Moberg, K., & Åsberg, M. (2012). Low CSF oxytocin reflects high intent in suicide attempters. *Psychoneuroendocrinology, 37*(4), 482–490.

Jokinen, J., Nordstrom, A. L., & Nordstrom, P. (2009). CSF 5-HIAA and DST non-suppression-orthogonal biologic risk factors for suicide in male mood disorder inpatients. *Psychiatry Research, 165*(1–2), 96–102.

Jollant, F., Lawrence, N. S., Olie, E., O'Daly, O., Malafosse, A., Courtet, P., & Phillips, M. L. (2010). Decreased activation of lateral orbitofrontal cortex during risky choices under uncertainty is associated with disadvantageous decision-making and suicidal behavior. *NeuroImage, 51*(3), 1275–1281.

Kaminsky, Z., Jones, I., Verma, R., Saleh, L., Trivedi, H., Guintivano, J., … Potash, J. B. (2015). DNA methylation and expression of KCNQ3 in bipolar disorder. *Bipolar Disorders, 17*(2), 150–159.

Labonté, B., Suderman, M., Maussion, G., Lopez, J. P., Navarro-Sánchez, L., Yerko, V., … Turecki, G. (2013). Genome-wide methylation changes in the brains of suicide completers. *American Journal of Psychiatry, 170*(5), 511–520.

Labonte, B., Yerko, V., Gross, J., Mechawar, N., Meaney, M. J., Szyf, M., & Turecki, G. (2012). Differential glucocorticoid receptor exon 1(B), 1(C), and 1(H) expression and methylation in suicide completers with a history of childhood abuse. *Biological Psychiatry, 72*(1), 41–48.

Lee, R., Ferris, C., Van de Kar, L. D., & Coccaro, E. F. (2009). Cerebrospinal fluid oxytocin, life history of aggression, and personality disorder. *Psychoneuroendocrinology, 34*(10), 1567–1573.

Lupien, S. J., McEwen, B. S., Gunnar, M. R., & Heim, C. (2009). Effects of stress throughout the lifespan on the brain, behaviour and cognition. *Nature Reviews Neuroscience, 10*(6), 434–445.

Mann, J. J. (2003). Neurobiology of suicidal behaviour. *Nature Reviews Neuroscience, 4*(10), 819–828.

Mann, J. J., & Currier, D. (2007). A review of prospective studies of biologic predictors of suicidal behavior in mood disorders. *Archives of Suicide Research, 11*(1), 3–16.

McGowan, P. O., Sasaki, A., D'Alessio, A. C., Dymov, S., Labonte, B., Szyf, M., … Meaney, M. J. (2009). Epigenetic regulation of the glucocorticoid receptor in human brain associates with childhood abuse. *Nature Neuroscience, 12*(3), 342–348.

Nemeroff, C. B., Owens, M. J., Bissette, G., Andorn, A. C., & Stanley, M. (1988). Reduced corticotropin releasing factor binding sites in the frontal cortex of suicide victims. *Archives of General Psychiatry, 45*(6), 577–579.

Neumann, I. D. (2009). The advantage of social living: Brain neuropeptides mediate the beneficial consequences of sex and motherhood. *Frontiers in Neuroendocrinology, 30*(4), 483–496.

Neumann, I. D., Krömer, S. A., Toschi, N., & Ebner, K. (2000). Brain oxytocin inhibits the (re) activity of the hypothalamo–pituitary–adrenal axis in male rats: Involvement of hypothalamic and limbic brain regions. *Regulatory Peptides, 96*(1–2), 31–38.

Neuringer, C. (1964). Rigid thinking in suicidal individuals. *Journal of Consulting Psychology, 28*, 54–58.

Niculescu, A. B., Levey, D. F., Phalen, P. L., Le-Niculescu, H., Dainton, H. D., Jain, N., … Salomon, D. R. (2015). Understanding and predicting suicidality using a combined genomic and clinical risk assessment approach. *Molecular Psychiatry, 20*(11), 1266–1285.

Nock, M. K., Borges, G., Bromet, E. J., Cha, C. B., Kessler, R. C., & Lee, S. (2008). Suicide and suicidal behavior. *Epidemiologic Reviews, 30*, 133–154.

Olff, M. (2012). Bonding after trauma: On the role of social support and the oxytocin system in traumatic stress. *European Journal of Psychotraumatology, 3*(1), 18597. https://doi.org/10.3402/ejpt.v3i0.18597

Opacka-Juffry, J., & Mohiyeddini, C. (2012). Experience of stress in childhood negatively correlates with plasma oxytocin concentration in adult men. *Stress, 15*(1), 1–10.

Oquendo, M. A., Sullivan, G. M., Sudol, K., Baca-Garcia, E., Stanley, B. H., Sublette, M. E., & Mann, J. J. (2014). Toward a biosignature for suicide. *The American Journal of Psychiatry, 171*(12), 1259–1277.

Perroud, N., Rutembesa, E., Paoloni-Giacobino, A., Mutabaruka, J., Mutesa, L., Stenz, L., … Karege, F. (2014). The Tutsi genocide and transgenerational transmission of maternal stress: Epigenetics and biology of the HPA axis. *The World Journal of Biological Psychiatry, 15*, 334.

Petersson, M., Hulting, A. L., & Uvnas-Moberg, K. (1999). Oxytocin causes a sustained decrease in plasma levels of corticosterone in rats. *Neuroscience Letters, 264*(1–3), 41–44.

Pfennig, A., Kunzel, H. E., Kern, N., Ising, M., Majer, M., Fuchs, B., … Binder, E. B. (2005). Hypothalamus-pituitary-adrenal system regulation and suicidal behavior in depression. *Biological Psychiatry, 57*(4), 336–342.

Pierrehumbert, B., Torrisi, R., Laufer, D., Halfon, O., Ansermet, F., & Beck Popovic, M. (2010). Oxytocin response to an experimental psychosocial challenge in adults exposed to traumatic experiences during childhood or adolescence. *Neuroscience, 166*(1), 168–177.

Policicchio, S., Washer, S., Viana, J., Iatrou, A., Burrage, J., Hannon, E., … Murphy, T. M. (2020). Genome-wide DNA methylation meta-analysis in the brains of suicide completers. *Translational Psychiatry, 10*(1), 1–13.

Rosell, D. R., & Siever, L. J. (2015). The neurobiology of aggression and violence. *CNS Spectrums, 20*(3), 254–279.

Roy, A., Gorodetsky, E., Yuan, Q., Goldman, D., & Enoch, M. A. (2010). Interaction of FKBP5, a stress-related gene, with childhood trauma increases the risk for attempting suicide. *Neuropsychopharmacology, 35*(8), 1674–1683.

Roy, B., Shelton, R. C., & Dwivedi, Y. (2017). DNA methylation and expression of stress related genes in PBMC of MDD patients with and without serious suicidal ideation. *Journal of Psychiatry Research, 89*, 115–124.

Seltzer, L. J., Ziegler, T., Connolly, M. J., Prososki, A. R., & Pollak, S. D. (2014). Stress-induced elevation of oxytocin in maltreated children: Evolution, neurodevelopment, and social behavior. *Child Development, 85*(2), 501–512.

Teicher, M. H., & Samson, J. A. (2013). Childhood maltreatment and psychopathology: A case for ecophenotypic variants as clinically and neurobiologically distinct subtypes. *American Journal of Psychiatry, 170*(10), 1114–1133.

Thompson, R. J., Parker, K. J., Hallmayer, J. F., Waugh, C. E., & Gotlib, I. H. (2011). Oxytocin receptor gene polymorphism (rs2254298) interacts with familial risk for psychopathology to predict symptoms of depression and anxiety in adolescent girls. *Psychoneuroendocrinology, 36*(1), 144–147.

Turecki, G. (2014). The molecular bases of the suicidal brain. *Nature Reviews Neuroscience, 15*(12), 802–816.

Turecki, G., & Brent, D. A. (2016). Suicide and suicidal behaviour. *Lancet, 387*, 1227. S0140-6736(15)00234-2.

Turecki, G., Ernst, C., Jollant, F., Labonte, B., & Mechawar, N. (2012). The neurodevelopmental origins of suicidal behavior. *Trends in Neurosciences, 35*(1), 14–23.

Turecki, G., Ota, V. K., Belangero, S. I., Jackowski, A., & Kaufman, J. (2014). Early life adversity, genomic plasticity, and psychopathology. *Lancet Psychiatry, 1*(6), 461–466.

van Heeringen, K., & Mann, J. J. (2014). The neurobiology of suicide. *Lancet Psychiatry, 1*(1), 63–72.

Veening, J. G., de Jong, T., & Barendregt, H. P. (2010). Oxytocin-messages via the cerebrospinal fluid: Behavioral effects; A review. *Physiology & Behavior, 101*(2), 193–210.

WHO. (2019). *Suicide*. Retrieved from https://www.who.int/news-room/fact-sheets/detail/suicide

Widom, C. S., Czaja, S. J., & Dutton, M. A. (2008). Childhood victimization and lifetime revictimization. *Child Abuse and Neglect, 32*(8), 785–796.

Windle, R. J., Kershaw, Y. M., Shanks, N., Wood, S. A., Lightman, S. L., & Ingram, C. D. (2004). Oxytocin attenuates stress-induced c-fos mRNA expression in specific forebrain regions associated with modulation of hypothalamo-pituitary-adrenal activity. *Journal of Neurosciece, 24*(12), 2974–2982.

Windle, R. J., Shanks, N., Lightman, S. L., & Ingram, C. D. (1997). Central oxytocin administration reduces stress-induced corticosterone release and anxiety behavior in rats. *Endocrinology, 138*(7), 2829–2834.

Yehuda, R., Daskalakis, N. P., Bierer, L. M., Bader, H. N., Klengel, T., Holsboer, F., & Binder, E. B. (2016). Holocaust exposure induced intergenerational effects on FKBP5 methylation. *Biological Psychiatry, 80*(5), 372–380.

Yrigollen, C. M., Han, S. S., Kochetkova, A., Babitz, T., Chang, J. T., Volkmar, F. R., ... Grigorenko, E. L. (2008). Genes controlling affiliative behavior as candidate genes for autism. *Biological Psychiatry, 63*(10), 911–916.

Chapter 2
Addressing Individualisation in Depression: Towards a Socially Informed Empowerment

Maria Orphanidou and Irini Kadianaki

Contents

Depression's popularity within the academic, clinical and public spheres is not novel. This popularity is largely attributed to depression's prevalence and vast reach on numerous aspects of life. Depression is a leading cause of disability worldwide (World Health Organization; WHO, 2020), with lifetime prevalence rate reaching 10.8% (Lim et al., 2018). It can inflict significant dysregulation over multiple areas of functioning including social roles and social functioning, academic and occupational performance, well-being and overall quality of life (Gotlib & Hammen, 2008). On a financial level, it is the costliest mental health disorder with costs exceeding 71 billion dollars (Dieleman et al., 2016). To minimise these burdens and subsequently improve people's lives, a significant amount of research has been devoted to understanding the factors involved in the emergence, perpetuation and treatment of depression (e.g. Dobson & Dozois, 2011; Kraus, Kadriu, Lanzenberger, Zarate, & Kasper, 2019).

Albeit this common underlying goal, several debates surround the nature and treatment of depression. One of the oldest debates is between theoretical approaches that adopt an individualistic understanding of depression and ones that emphasise its social underpinnings. The former are aligned with medical conceptualisations,

M. Orphanidou (✉) · I. Kadianaki
Department of Psychology, University of Cyprus, Nicosia, Cyprus
e-mail: orphanidou.maria@ucy.ac.cy; kadianaki.irini@ucy.ac.cy

© Springer Nature Switzerland AG 2021   17
C. Charis, G. Panayiotou (eds.), *Depression Conceptualization and Treatment*,
https://doi.org/10.1007/978-3-030-68932-2_2

which highlight the role of biomarkers, neurotransmitters and genes, as well as psychological conceptualisations that emphasise cognitive, affective and behavioural processes (Dobson & Dozois, 2011). Within such approaches, treatment is mainly centred on the individual who is expected to manage symptoms either via medication or psychotherapy (Gotlib & Hammen, 2008). In contrast, theoretical approaches of a social basis stress the role of wider social factors (e.g. gender, race, socioeconomic status, unemployment, access to care; Assari, 2017) while criticising the individualisation of depression for being imbued with neoliberal ideas of self-governance and individual responsibility (Philip, 2009). Specifically, they argue that under the pretences of self-improvement and autonomy, individuals are held accountable for things that lie outside their immediate control (Brijnath & Antoniades, 2018). For instance, findings suggest that individuals are treated as the only ones responsible for overcoming depression, despite its evident socioeconomic causes (Teghtsoonian, 2009). Be that as it may, not all researchers view patient accountability in the treatment process as problematic. In fact, some argue that encouraging patients to take control of treatment and subsequently their health is a positive development, since it can facilitate empowerment (Duggal, 2019; Houle et al., 2016; van Grieken, van Tricht, Koeter, van den Brink, & Schene, 2018). From this perspective, patient accountability is viewed in terms of empowerment and discussed as a positive outcome that leads to reduced depressive symptoms and increased well-being (Hart Abney, Lusk, Hovermale, & Melnyk, 2019).

While one approach accentuates the benefits of agency and active patient involvement (i.e. patients showing initiative and making decisions relating to the treatment process; Duggal, 2019), the other maintains a critical stance towards self-responsibilisation and the individualisation of depression (Philip, 2009). The seemingly irreconcilable nature of empowerment and individualisation discourses has resulted in a dichotomic relationship, which has led to dead-end in the literature examining the individual's role in depression. As we discuss below, albeit the genuine risk of individualising depression that is linked to empowerment practices, the unquestionable endorsement of the critical individualisation discourse runs the risk of victimising patients and denying agency. Thus, it is our belief that the way forwards is not to merely illuminate the pitfalls of depression's individualisation but, rather, to empower individuals in a way that does not overwhelm them and ceases to feed into the growing individualisation of the condition. We argue that to achieve this, researchers need to open up to the possibility of a dialectic relationship between the two discourses. Currently, only few authors point to the interconnection of these discourses, suggesting that the two may not be as irreconcilable as they appear. For example, Rivest and Moreau (2015) call for a shift from individual empowerment alone to the inclusion of community and organisational empowerment. They argue that this can achieve a balance between the individualism of current practices and the need for social interventions. O'Connor and Nagel (2017) also critique the dichotomy by proposing that self-improvement is not necessarily linked to neoliberalism but is affected by social factors too. Particularly, they give evidence for relational rather than individual factors being the driving force of neuro-enhancement.

Given findings that point to the central role of the individual in the aetiology (e.g. individual causal factors such as weakness of character and personality traits; Cook & Wang, 2011) and treatment of depression (e.g. self-management; Duggal, 2019), we argue that overcoming the current blockade may be of particular importance for depression. In this chapter, we aim to illuminate this dead-end and explore whether finding a way towards a socially informed empowerment that does not come at the expense of agency is possible. The chapter opens with an overview of the rise of individual factors in depression and how this rise is understood by the two discourses. Next, using data from our research on the social representations (Moscovici, 1961/2008) and experiences of depression in patients, the need for addressing the strongly individualised nature of depression while maintaining agency is discussed. The chapter closes with implications of this approach and suggestions for moving forwards.

2.1 The Individual in the Spotlight of Depression

When it comes to understanding and treating psychological disorders, the biopsychosocial model (Engel, 1977) is among the most popular frameworks. Although the model places equal emphasis on biological (e.g. genetics, neurotransmitters, increased reactivity), psychological (e.g. cognitive and affective processes, personality traits) and social (e.g. relationships, socioeconomic factors, culture, unemployment) aspects of psychological disorders, ever since the "decade of the brain", a shift has been noted. In comparison to individual aspects, namely, biological and to a lesser extent psychological factors, social aspects are somewhat marginalised (Compton & Shim, 2015).

In the case of depression, social factors such as poverty, low socioeconomic status and unemployment are not necessarily marginalised, but instead treated as taken-for-granted kind of variables (Compton & Shim, 2015) to explain vulnerability towards depression (e.g. gender, traumatic experiences, socioeconomic background; Gotlib & Hammen, 2008). When it comes to treating depression, attention is mainly turned to individual factors leaving social ones partially addressed (Cosgrove & Karter, 2018). Particularly, the social factors targeted are usually found within the immediate environment of the individual; hence, they are things that can be changed by the individual (e.g. social skills, involvement in social activities; Gotlib & Hammen, 2008). Surprisingly, even when wider social factors like unemployment and poverty are addressed, responsibility for tackling these factors falls on the individual and not on sociopolitical agents or the state (Teghtsoonian, 2009). Additionally, there is an increasing literature encouraging individuals to assert control over treatment (Duggal, 2019; Hart Abney et al., 2019). This control may be exercised through several means, including implementing critical lifestyle changes to self-manage depression (e.g. exercise, healthy diet, use of self-help books) and assuming responsibility to seek professional help (Duggal, 2019). Therefore, once again, emphasis is placed on the individual and his/her capacities rather than the role of wider social influences.

Given the information discussed, it is evident that when it comes to depression and its treatment, the individual has moved to the spotlight. This placement has resulted in a growing debate whether such an individualistic path is benefiting or hindering patients. As we discuss below, researchers from the field of empowerment favour the former, whereas researchers who are sceptical about the growing indi-vidualisation of depression align with the latter.

2.1.1 Empowering Individuals to Reclaim Control over Depression

Despite its emergence in the early 1950s, over the past decade or so, the concept of empowerment, and its application in clinical settings relating to physical and mental health, has attracted a lot of attention (Anderson & Funnell, 2010; WHO, 2010). Rooted in principles of autonomy, self-determination and individuals' ability to make the right choices for their well-being (McCarley, 2009), empowerment was introduced by Rappaport (1981) in an effort to move beyond the medical paternal-ism encountered in the healthcare. Via emphasising the need for the active involve-ment of patients in decisions concerning their health and via facilitating individuals to take control (WHO, 2010), the concept of patient empowerment led to a radical restructuring of the interactions between patients, health professionals and the healthcare system (Fitzsimons & Fuller, 2002). Particularly, patients are no longer treated as passive recipients of expert knowledge but as active agents within the treatment process.

Although empowerment is a concept that cuts across multiple levels of a society, namely, the individual, community and organisational/structural levels (WHO, 2010), in the domain of mental health, attention is mainly turned to the individual level (Rivest & Moreau, 2015). Individual or patient empowerment is a multifaceted construct, which refers to higher confidence in one's abilities (self-efficacy), an increased sense of mastery and control over situations that affect an individual's life (self-determination), self-acceptance and a positive view of self (self-esteem), as well as a drive to achieve one's goals and improve overall well-being (Zimmerman & Rappaport, 1988). It is both a process (i.e. the process through which an indi-vidual develops the aforementioned qualities) and an outcome (i.e. the achievement of these qualities; Fitzsimons & Fuller, 2002). Further, it has been linked to better health outcomes, treatment adherence and higher quality of life (WHO, 2010). Therefore, it is not surprising why researchers advocate for the empowerment of patients in physical and mental health contexts, regardless of their diagnosis (e.g. Anderson & Funnell, 2010; WHO, 2010).

The application of empowerment principles in the treatment of depression appears to be fitting for many reasons. Firstly, the concept of power, or lack thereof, has an intricate relationship with depression. Even nowadays, depression is associated with beliefs about weakness of character not only within lay discourses (Cook & Wang, 2011), but most importantly within patient discourses (Rungreangkulkij, Kotnara, Kittiwatanapaisan, & Arunpongpaisal, 2019). By incorporating empowerment principles in the treatment process, such misconceptions and stigmatising beliefs can possibly be addressed. Through empowerment, patients can uncover the power they believe they lack and achieve personal and clinical recovery (Duggal, 2019). The former refers to the ability to lead a fulfilled and meaningful life even in cases where symptoms persist, whereas the latter to the depletion of clinical symptoms (Slade, 2009).

The experience of depression has also been linked to loss of self-control over cognitive, emotional and behavioural aspects (Rungreangkulkij et al., 2019). Empowerment enables patients to develop confidence in their abilities to manage symptoms and regain control of their life; thus, it may be particularly fitting for treating depression (Duggal, 2019). Lastly, in cases of chronic conditions or ones that are highly recurrent, such as depression (Burcusa & Iacono, 2007), the empowerment of patients, and the subsequent increase in the self-management of their health, can contribute in reducing the strains exerted by depression on the healthcare system. As patients learn to self-regulate milder symptoms with no or minimal input from professionals, they are able to maintain positive treatment outcomes longer, and it minimises the utilisation of the healthcare system (Duggal, 2019).

Individual empowerment can be achieved with or without professional guidance. According to the WHO (2010, p. 3), the aim of patient empowerment is to help individuals "gain understanding, voice and influence over decisions that affect their lives". This aim governs all professional mental health practices. Meanwhile, the self-management of depression without professional guidance is also aligned with principles of empowerment, as individuals develop autonomy and use available information to choose between treatment options, based on what they believe is better suited for them (van Grieken et al., 2018).

Claims for a positive impact of empowerment on depression are supported in the literature. Findings from patients across 20 European countries diagnosed with depression or bipolar disorder illustrated that higher levels of empowerment were linked with significantly lower levels of self-stigma (Brohan et al., 2011). Such findings echo evidence for an inverse relationship between empowerment and self-stigmatisation (Rüsch, Lieb, Bohus, & Corrigan, 2006). In Sweden, a study on unemployed individuals diagnosed with depression or bipolar disorder illustrated that the implementation of an empowerment-based intervention to facilitate individuals' efforts to return to work increased empowerment levels and quality of life while decreasing the severity of depressive symptoms (Johanson & Bejerholm, 2017). These positive outcomes were maintained up to a year later (Porter & Bejerholm, 2018). Further, empowerment programmes show promising results in reducing depressive symptoms and increasing well-being in people of different ages diagnosed with depression, including young adults (Hart Abney et al., 2019) and elders (Mobaraki, Kamali, & Farhodi, 2013). Despite the auspicious literature examined illuminating the relevance of empowerment in the treatment of depression, the use of empowerment principles in therapeutic interventions does not remain unchallenged.

2.1.2   Overwhelmed Individuals and the Individualisation of Depression

Coming from a more critical perspective on mental health, several researchers remain sceptical about the impact of patient empowerment on the basis of its individualistic nature (Beck & Beck-Gernsheim, 2002; Nagel, 2010), which they view as a dealignment from the multilevel origins of the construct (Rivest & Moreau, 2015). Specifically, they argue that empowerment has been imbued with the individualistic ethos of modern societies, an outcome which runs the risk of overwhelming individuals by assigning responsibility even for things outside their control (Nagel, 2010). Individualisation can be described as the process of shifting attention inwards, that is, to understand different phenomena, attention is turned to individual factors, whereas the contribution of the social context is largely ignored (Beck & Beck-Gernsheim, 2002). Individualisation is also linked to self-governance. Particularly, the desire to exert self-control and lead autonomous lives is strongly engraved in Western cultures (Beck & Beck-Gernsheim, 2002). In line with principles of neoliberalism, active citizenship and moral responsibility, the strive for autonomy, self-improvement and self-actualisation is gaining momentum across Western societies (Cosgrove & Karter, 2018). This individualistic mentality governs all domains of human functioning, including physical and mental health (Crawford, 2006; O'Connor, Rees, & Joffe, 2012), which have become another project that individuals need to work on unremittingly (O'Connor et al., 2012). In the case of depression, the emphasis on individual aetiological factors (e.g. genetics, cognitive processes, personality traits, serotonin levels) and the accentuated role of the individual in the treatment process are clear examples of individualisation (Philip, 2009; Teghtsoonian, 2009). In line with this neoliberal strive for self-enhancement, individuals are also encouraged to self-manage their depression using the appropriate professional or non-professional means (Duggal, 2019).

Thus, critics are concerned with whether assuming a leading role in the treatment process is an individual's choice or responsibility (Teghtsoonian, 2009). Some even argue that depression has been transformed into a moral problem that individuals need to overcome, if they wish to conform to Westernised principles of active and responsible citizens (Philip, 2009). At a first glance, such an individualistic, neoliberal approach may sound promising as individuals are seemingly free to decide if they want to look after their health or not. Yet, on a closer examination, the dangers of self-responsibilisation and self-blame are illuminated (Cosgrove & Karter, 2018; Teghtsoonian, 2009). Individuals are expected to look after their health, become the optimal version of themselves and thus reduce unwarranted burdens to the health-care system (Cosgrove & Karter, 2018; Teghtsoonian, 2009). Having the opportunity to self-manage depression yet choosing not to can be perceived as a failure to do the responsible thing. Hence, individuals may be harshly judged by others and themselves for their inaction (Esposito & Perez, 2014; Nagel, 2010). This judgement is exercised even in cases where depression is clearly attributed to social factors that are outside the individual's control (Teghtsoonian, 2009). In this respect, assuming responsibility for the treatment of depression is no longer a choice but rather an obligation. Thus, failure to oblige is constructed as an individual failure, which is attributed to lack of incentive, irresponsibility and/or some kind of individual pathology (Beck & Beck-Gernsheim, 2002; Cosgrove & Karter, 2018).

The individualisation of depression is also linked to the marginalisation of social factors in understanding and treating depression (Brijnath & Antoniades, 2018; Philip, 2009; Rivest & Moreau, 2015). By attributing it primarily on factors located in an individual's body, depression is constructed as a problem of the individual. Hence, responsibility for addressing it also falls on the individual (Esposito & Perez, 2014; Teghtsoonian, 2009). This downplay of the social context runs the risk of increasing victim-blaming and stigmatisation, both from others and the self. Philip (2009) argues that individuals become increasingly convinced that the emergence of depression is somehow their fault and subsequently their responsibility. By shifting responsibility to individuals alone, they become less likely to challenge wider social injustices (e.g. unemployment, exploitation of labour, poor living conditions) that may be linked to their suffering (Philip, 2009; Summerfield, 2008). Consequently, it can be claimed that rather than empowered, individuals are gradually being overwhelmed as they shoulder a much larger share of responsibility than they should.

The empowerment discourse is also criticised for its culture-bound applicability. Research suggests that the application of neoliberal principles of self-improvement among people with non-Western cultural backgrounds may be ill-suited and inappropriate (Summerfield, 2008). In fact, the widespread use of Western approaches is critiqued for medical imperialism, and researchers call for culturally sensitive treatment options (Dowrick, 2013; Summerfield, 2013). Independent of the cultural background, health professionals caution that for many individuals taking the treatment reins may be overwhelming, since they often arrive at therapy as a last resort, feeling lost and ineffective (Rivest & Moreau, 2015).

Paradoxically, the interventions meant to liberate and empower patients run the risk of overwhelming and stigmatising the people they aspire to help (Philip, 2009). To address these shortcomings, researchers urge for a powershift from the individual to the social via targeting the social determinants of depression (i.e. the conditions in which people are born into, live, work and age that affect their well-being; Shim et al., 2014). Using data from our qualitative research on understandings and the experience of depression among Greek-Cypriots patients, below we show that these risks expand from the academic realm to that of daily life. The extracts presented below originate from a larger project exploring the social representations (Moscovici, 1961/2008) of depression within the Greek-Cypriot press (Orphanidou & Kadianaki, 2020), public and patients. The data were collected through eight semi-structured individual interviews with patients between the ages of 16 and 80.

Our aim here is not to analyse the data but to use them as illustrations for the afore-mentioned discourses and their critiques.

2.2   The Need for a Socially Informed Empowerment

The exploration of patient discourses corroborates the growing individualisation of depression and its adverse impact on patients. Data suggest that patients represent depression as an issue of the individual. For example, in the extract[1] below, Thodoris discounts the contribution of psychosocial factors such as the familial environment in the aetiology of depression and assumes total responsibility for its emergence, perpetuation and treatment:

> Thodoris (M, 16–20 years old): [Depression] was due to my stupid [reactions] of [over-thinking] and anxiety, (…) and my personality traits. (…) Many times, I create problems for myself on my own to be honest. It is no one else's fault. (…) [The psychiatrist and psychologist] believed that my family environment had an effect. The situations that I experienced at home. The fights, the noise, the yelling, my uncle's drug use. I wouldn't say it's [their] fault. (…) I believe it's my problem, I am responsible.

In line with critics of individualisation, Thodoris's extract illustrates how the transformation of depression into an individual issue could cultivate a negative view of the self. Particularly, it illuminates the over-responsibilisation of the self in relation to the aetiology and treatment of depression, which in turn encourages self-blaming and self-stigmatisation (Philip, 2009).

Interestingly, the construction of depression as an individual issue is so strong that it persists even in cases where participants acknowledge the role of the psychosocial context in triggering depression. In his interview, Alexandros attributes the emergence of depression to the chronic bullying he experienced throughout school and his lack of friends, whereas Melina talks about the role of a traumatic event she experienced and her family's financial troubles. Regardless, in the following extracts, both participants draft strong links between depression and individual causal factors, namely, personality traits and cognitive processes; hence, treatment is perceived as their responsibility alone:

> Alexandros (M, 16-20 years old): You put yourself in a prison, in a box, so I believe [depression] is a torture. Um, you imprison yourself on your own, no one else is putting you there, and you create things with your thoughts, and the only one responsible for this situation is you. (…) No one can help you if you don't want to help yourself.

> Melina (F, 40-55 years old): The weak ones, the sensitive ones [are affected more by depression]. (…) I was a weak character. (…) You need strength. Maybe you acquire this strength because you are suffering? And you say [to yourself] that you need to do something, you

---

[1] "" indicates an extract from the data; [ ] indicates an addition of text for explanation purposes; (…) indicates omitted text that is irrelevant to the analysis; to protect anonymity, pseudonyms are used for all participants.

can't stay like this. (...) I told myself that I will fight [depression] on my own. (...) If [the pills] help me and I help myself, I will make it.

What is noteworthy is how deeply internalised is the idea that depression is an individual issue. Even when factors extending beyond the individual are recognised, the sense of individual responsibility, particularly over treatment, remains unwavering. In a way, self-responsibilisation is understood as a fundamental part of treatment. Therefore, it appears that patient discourses do indeed reflect the shortcomings of individualisation discussed above.

For most participants, assuming responsibility for the treatment process is also linked to a sense of empowerment. Despite the uncertainty regarding the origins of her new founded strength, Melina's extract supports claims that patient accountability is to some extent linked to empowerment. Similarly, Konstantina's extract on the positive outcomes of having depression is a clear example of patient empowerment cultivated in psychotherapy:

> Konstantina (F, 25–35 years old): Psychotherapy. [It's] when you discover your strengths and that it's okay for others not to like you. [You] learn things, [you] change, [you] begin to love yourself. [You] work on yourself and to get to know yourself. (...) Little by little, you discover your strengths. Umm, not only that I can do this activity but that I can also start one that I never imagined I could do, and I can actually do it well. You get out of your comfort zone, um, that you will handle everything alone. And you begin to ask for help. (...) I managed to get out of [depression] so [it means] that I am strong.

Konstantina describes with satisfaction and pride a number of individual accomplishments that she achieved in handling depression. Interestingly, asking for help and not depending on one's own is one of them. In her words, there is a sense of empowerment, which in this case is a process that involves both the self and the immediate social context. Still, the strongly individualising nature of her discourse remains prominent as the spotlight is primarily on her. This individualisation becomes even more apparent when the disproportionate involvement of social factors in the treatment of depression is examined. Although Konstantina considers the financial crisis and her subsequent loss of employment as key aetiological factors for her depression, the role of the social context in the treatment process is restricted to the immediate environment, whereas the contribution of the wider social context is non-existent. This restriction was evident in all of the interviews conducted.

The data examined illuminate the validity of the individualisation critique. As we have shown, the belief that depression is exclusively the responsibility of the individual has become so deeply internalised that it remains unchallenged among patients. Although we concur with critics warning against the pitfalls of individualisation, we argue that a total and unquestionable endorsement of its critique leads to an impasse in the treatment of depression. Specifically, we propose that the shift from patient empowerment to social determinants alone possibly hinders individual change and dealing with depression since patients are treated as victims of the wider social circumstances. Such victimisation denies agency, places patients in a passive position and is linked to poorer mental health outcome (Vitz, 2005). On the other hand, the overemphasis on individual factors noted in current practices may offer a sense of empowerment, yet it appears to be at the expense of the social factors involved in depression and, most importantly, with the cost of overwhelming individuals. Consequently, researchers and patients alike seem to be "trapped" in a dead-end that one way or another hinders the treatment of depression. Coming from a dialectic standpoint, we recognise both the relevance of empowerment and the validity of the individualisation critique in depression. Hence, moving forwards, we suggest the inclusion of more social aspects in the understanding and treatment of depression is essential. However, we argue that it needs to be done in a way that maintains agency, does not hinder individual change and does not victimise patients. As we discuss below, we urge for a more socially informed empowerment on all three levels.

2.3   Towards a Socially Informed Empowerment

Nowadays, empowerment is understood as a highly individualised construct, but if its theoretical roots are examined, its close ties with the wider sociocultural context are evident (Fitzsimons & Fuller, 2002; Rivest & Moreau, 2015). As Fitzsimons and Fuller (2002) note, empowerment is neither a trait nor a tangible entity that can be passed from one individual to the next. Rather, it develops based on the kind of interactions individuals have with their immediate and wider social contexts (e.g. family, friends, community, work, culture). Growing up in a validating and encouraging familial context, being part of a community that promotes participation in community activities and a sense of community belonging and living in a society that respects human rights, battles unemployment and poverty and encourages equal access to care are just few examples of how one's context could enable empowerment development and well-being (WHO, 2010). Interestingly, such changes in the immediate and wider social context promote empowerment both on the corresponding level (e.g. changes encouraging a sense of community belonging facilitate empowerment of the community; WHO, 2010) and the individual level of empowerment too (Corrigan, 2002; WHO, 2010).

   Yet in current practices, this understanding seems to be marginalised in favour of the individual. Even though the neoliberal ethos and the strong principles of self-governance encountered in Western cultures offer one explanation for this marginalisation (Esposito & Perez, 2014), we propose that practical difficulties may play a role too. Particularly, to facilitate community and organisational empowerment, wider sociopolitical agents and resources need to be mobilised (Shim et al., 2014). However, such changes are not easily enforced. Numerous agents are involved, and oftentimes, a significant amount of time may pass before their implementation. So, it is possible that in an attempt to compensate for these barriers and offer a more immediate solution in the treatment of depression, mental health professionals focus on individual factors, which are more easily amenable.

   Thus far, the need for an ideological shift away from the neoliberalism of Western cultures and biomedical understandings of health/illness has been reiterated by many critics (e.g. Cosgrove & Karter, 2018; Esposito & Perez, 2014). To bring back the social in health, critics urge for interventions promoting community and organisational empowerment (Rivest & Moreau, 2015). For instance, calls have been made for public health campaigns targeting the social determinants of health (Smith et al., 2014), community programmes that support the treatment of mental illness via helping individuals develop skills, finding employment and peer support (Brijnath & Antoniades, 2018) as well as policy changes that reduce stigma and discrimination, promote patient rights and reinstate the share of responsibility for depression that belongs to the state (Compton & Shim, 2015; WHO, 2010). Although such suggestions work towards changing the cultural ideology driving the individualisation of depression, the practical difficulties hindering their implementation remain unaddressed. Perhaps this is why albeit years of research, attempts to minimise the individualisation of depression have limited success. Hence, we propose that research on interventions stimulating community and organisational empowerment should also explore ways of minimising practical difficulties.

Concurrently, research should expand beyond the community and organisational levels. Even though these levels appear to be more compatible with the aforementioned ideological shift, we argue that only when this shift is implemented on the individual level of empowerment too, we can escape the current blockade. Thus, we urge for a move towards a socially informed individual empowerment. To achieve this, we propose that in therapeutic settings, professionals should aim for the incorporation of more social factors, particularly the wider social determinants of health, in understandings of depression. At the same time, the role of wider sociopolitical agents in the treatment of depression should be explicitly recognised too. While patients may not be at a position to directly manipulate these wider social factors, professionals should avoid emphasising only patient empowerment. We argue that given the era of the individual that we live in, the need for reminding patients about the role of the wider social context in conjunction with empowerment interventions is essential. It is our belief that such changes, in addition to a broader ideological shift, could slowly encourage a change in patient's beliefs about treatment responsibility. Hence, it can facilitate a socially informed patient empowerment that safeguards patient agency and reduces individualisation.

2.4 Conclusion

The individual's role in the aetiology and treatment of depression has become the bone of contention among researchers favouring patient empowerment and ones criticising individualisation. While both discourses raise valid points that are particularly relevant in depression, as we have shown, treating them as irreconcilable discourses has led to a dead-end. Rather than choosing between the two, we have argued for a shift towards a more socially informed empowerment that acknowledges the role of the social context and safeguards patient agency. Although we offer some suggestions of how this shift may be achieved, we recognise the need for further research in this area. Thus, future research should aim to examine the implementation and implications of this socially informed empowerment.

References

Anderson, R. M., & Funnell, M. M. (2010). Patient empowerment: Myths and misconceptions. *Patient Education and Counseling, 79*(3), 277–282.

Assari, S. (2017). Social determinants of depression: The intersections of race, gender, and socioeconomic status. *Brain Sciences, 7*(12), 156–167.

Beck, U., & Beck-Gernsheim, E. (2002). *Individualization: Institutionalized individualism and its social and political consequences.* London: SAGE.

Brijnath, B., & Antoniades, J. (2018). Beyond patient culture: Filtering cultural presentations of depression through structural terms. *Critical Public Health, 28*(2), 237–247.

Brohan, E., Gauci, D., Sartorius, N., Thornicroft, G., & GAMIAN–Europe Study Group. (2011). Self-stigma, empowerment and perceived discrimination among people with bipolar disorder or depression in 13 European countries: The GAMIAN–Europe study. *Journal of Affective Disorders, 129*(1–3), 56–63.

Burcusa, S. L., & Iacono, W. G. (2007). Risk for recurrence in depression. *Clinical Psychology Review, 27*(8), 959–985.

Compton, M. T., & Shim, R. S. (2015). The social determinants of mental health. *Focus, 13*(4), 419–425.

Cook, T. M., & Wang, J. (2011). Causation beliefs and stigma against depression: Results from a population-based study. *Journal of Affective Disorders, 133*(1–2), 86–92.

Corrigan, P. W. (2002). Empowerment and serious mental illness: Treatment partnerships and community opportunities. *Psychiatric Quarterly, 73*(3), 217–228.

Cosgrove, L., & Karter, J. M. (2018). The poison in the cure: Neoliberalism and contemporary movements in mental health. *Theory & Psychology, 28*(5), 669–683.

Crawford, R. (2006). Health as a meaningful social practice. *Health, 10*(4), 401–420.

Dieleman, J. L., Baral, R., Birger, M., Bui, A. L., Bulchis, A., Chapin, A., … Lavado, R. (2016). US spending on personal health care and public health, 1996-2013. *JAMA, 316*(24), 2627–2646.

Dobson, K. S., & Dozois, D. J. (Eds.). (2011). *Risk factors in depression.* London: Elsevier.

Dowrick, C. (2013). Depression as a culture-bound syndrome: Implications for primary care. *British Journal of General Practice, 63*(610), 229–230.

Duggal, H. S. (2019). Self-management of depression: Beyond the medical model. *The Permanente Journal, 23*, 18–295. https://doi.org/10.7812/TPP/18-295

Engel, G. L. (1977). The need for a new medical model: A challenge for biomedicine. *Science, 196*(4286), 129–136.

Esposito, L., & Perez, F. M. (2014). Neoliberalism and the commodification of mental health. *Humanity and Society, 38*(4), 414–442.

Fitzsimons, S., & Fuller, R. (2002). Empowerment and its implications for clinical practice in mental health: A review. *Journal of Mental Health, 11*(5), 481–499.

Gotlib, I. H., & Hammen, C. L. (Eds.). (2008). *Handbook of depression* (2nd ed.). New York, NY: Guilford Press.

Hart Abney, B. G., Lusk, P., Hovermale, R., & Melnyk, B. M. (2019). Decreasing depression and anxiety in college youth using the Creating Opportunities for Personal Empowerment Program (COPE). *Journal of the American Psychiatric Nurses Association, 25*(2), 89–98.

Houle, J., Gauvin, G., Collard, B., Meunier, S., Frasure-Smith, N., Lespérance, F., … Lambert, J. (2016). Empowering adults in recovery from depression: A community-based self-management group program. *Canadian Journal of Community Mental Health, 35*(2), 55–68.

Johanson, S., & Bejerholm, U. (2017). The role of empowerment and quality of life in depression severity among unemployed people with affective disorders receiving mental healthcare. *Disability and Rehabilitation, 39*(18), 1807–1813.

Kraus, C., Kadriu, B., Lanzenberger, R., Zarate, C. A., Jr., & Kasper, S. (2019). Prognosis and improved outcomes in major depression: A review. *Translational Psychiatry, 9*(1), 1–17.

Lim, G. Y., Tam, W. W., Lu, Y., Ho, C. S., Zhang, M. W., & Ho, R. C. (2018). Prevalence of depression in the community from 30 countries between 1994 and 2014. *Scientific Reports, 8*(1), 2861–2870.

McCarley, P. (2009). Patient empowerment and motivational interviewing: Engaging patients to self-manage their own care. *Nephrology Nursing Journal, 36*(4), 409–413.

Mobaraki, H., Kamali, M., & Farhodi, F. (2013). The effect of empowerment programs on geriatric depression in daily rehabilitation Farzanegan center of khorramabad city. *Modern Rehabilitation, 6*(4), 65–70.

Moscovici, S. (2008). *Psychoanalysis: Its image and its public*. Cambridge: Polity Press. (Original work published in 1961).

Nagel, S. K. (2010). Too much of a good thing? Enhancement and the burden of self-determination. *Neuroethics, 3*(2), 109–119.

O'Connor, C., & Nagel, S. K. (2017). Neuro-enhancement practices across the lifecourse: Exploring the roles of relationality and individualism. *Frontiers in Sociology, 2*, 1.

O'Connor, C., Rees, G., & Joffe, H. (2012). Neuroscience in the public sphere. *Neuron, 74*(2), 220–226.

Orphanidou, M., & Kadianaki, I. (2020). Between medicalisation and normalisation: Antithetical representations of depression in the Greek-Cypriot press in times of financial crisis. *Health (London, England), 24*, 403. https://doi.org/10.1177/1363459318804579

Philip, B. (2009). Analysing the politics of self-help books on depression. *Journal of Sociology, 45*(2), 151–168.

Porter, S., & Bejerholm, U. (2018). The effect of individual enabling and support on empowerment and depression severity in persons with affective disorders: Outcome of a randomized control trial. *Nordic Journal of Psychiatry, 72*(4), 259–267.

Rappaport, J. (1981). In praise of paradox: A social policy of empowerment over prevention. *American Journal of Community Psychology, 9*, 1–25.

Rivest, M. P., & Moreau, N. (2015). Between emancipatory practice and disciplinary interventions: Empowerment and contemporary social normativity. *The British Journal of Social Work, 45*(6), 1855–1870.

Rungreangkulkij, S., Kotnara, I., Kittiwatanapaisan, W., & Arunpongpaisal, S. (2019). Loss of control: Experiences of depression in Thai men. *Walailak Journal of Science and Technology (WJST), 16*(4), 265–274.

Rüsch, N., Lieb, K., Bohus, M., & Corrigan, P. W. (2006). Self-stigma, empowerment, and perceived legitimacy of discrimination among women with mental illness. *Psychiatric Services, 57*(3), 399–402.

Shim, R., Koplan, C., Langheim, F. J., Manseau, M. W., Powers, R. A., & Compton, M. T. (2014). The social determinants of mental health: An overview and call to action. *Psychiatric Annals, 44*(1), 22–26.

Slade, M. (2009). The contribution of mental health services to recovery. *Journal of Mental Health, 18*(5), 367–371. https://doi.org/10.3109/09638230903191256

Summerfield, D. (2008). How scientifically valid is the knowledge base of global mental health? *BMJ, 336*(7651), 992–994.

Summerfield, D. (2013). "Global mental health" is an oxymoron and medical imperialism. *BMJ, 346*, f3509.

Teghtsoonian, K. (2009). Depression and mental health in neoliberal times: A critical analysis of policy and discourse. *Social Science & Medicine, 69*(1), 28–35.

van Grieken, R. A., van Tricht, M. J., Koeter, M., van den Brink, W., & Schene, A. H. (2018). The use and helpfulness of self-management strategies for depression: The experiences of patients. *PLoS One, 13*(10), e0206262. https://doi.org/10.1371/journal.pone.0206262

Vitz, P. (2005). Psychology in recovery. *First Things, 151*(1), 17–21.

World Health Organization. (2010). *User empowerment in mental health: A statement by the WHO Regional Office for Europe - Empowerment is not a destination, but a journey.* Copenhagen: WHO. Regional Office for Europe.

World Health Organization. (2020, 30 January). *Depression.* Retrieved from https://www.who.int/news-room/fact-sheets/detail/depression

Zimmerman, M. A., & Rappaport, J. (1988). Citizen participation, perceived control, and psychological empowerment. *American Journal of Community Psychology, 16*(5), 725–750.

Chapter 3
Psychodynamics in Depression: A Short Case. Symptom Formation, Mentalization, Symptom Solution

Andreas Bilger

Case A 40-year-old woman was assigned to me by her physician, as she had been suffering from depression for a long time without help from medication and behavioral advice by her doctor, with whom she had had good and trusting contact for a long time …

Now, after four psychotherapy sessions over 2 months she felt a significant change in her mood and depressive symptoms, and developed changing and more efficient attitudes in parts of her life, especially in her marriage and in her professional field.

The example may show that even severe and persistent complaints may be influenced by psychotherapeutic intervention, even within a short time, even if other attempts did not succeed, e.g., therapy in a psychosomatic unit, in-patient treatment on a ward.

The woman has been suffering from depression, chronic discontent, and a kind of pathological jealousy toward her partner, her former lover, and now her husband, for 10 years.

Early in the interview it became obvious that the patient was full of complaints and tended to turn every lamentation into self-complaints and self-accusations, leading to a circle of self-dissatisfaction, depressed temper, and anger in her voice, the current atmosphere, and in relationships.

Now that a dream of being married to her friend, a wish she had had for a long time, had been fulfilled, she had been suffering from permanent anxiety that the marriage would be wrecked by her guilt (by her jealousy), and her depressed tension is often so strong that she has suicidal thoughts.

When she was speaking, I could clearly feel the tension she lived with in her marriage. To be more precise: she seemed not to be allowed to have this

A. Bilger (✉)
University Ulm, Ulm, Germany
e-mail: andreas.bilger@uni-ulm.de

© Springer Nature Switzerland AG 2021
C. Charis, G. Panayiotou (eds.), *Depression Conceptualization and Treatment*,
https://doi.org/10.1007/978-3-030-68932-2_3

consciousness about her tensions, as at any moment, when she was beginning to shout about the attitudes of her beloved but apparently rather imperious husband, she was used to immediately turning the anger, rage, and disappointment toward herself. As she was quite full of spirit and not a typically passive depressed woman, and as she repeated this self-accusing behavior during the interview, this tension and anger constituted a major topic in the relationship.

If we followed naively the many and various problems, complaints, and life events that the patient demonstrated and talked about during the first session, we would soon have the depressing impression that there have been a variety of unsolvable conflicts and anxieties since early childhood that have developed and followed one another, which would be hard to change, even with intensive long-term psychotherapy.

Clinical theory and experience suggest that depression and pathological self-dissatisfaction may be associated with disguised, unconscious aggressive activity and guilty feelings or fantasies. This seems to be of special interest when the depressive complaints occur paradoxically within positive life changes and/or relief from "stress." These guilty feelings are accompanied by a subliminal fear of one's own activity that appears obvious to others from the outside, and aggressivity (which is frequently there to excess). Of course, this fear blocks all of one's own initiatives and natural joy of life, a fact that leads to the typical clinical expression of depressed patients: a passive, ambivalent impression, powerless but full of tension.

From this point of view, in the first interview, besides and in spite of the confusing variety of life events, sorrows, and preoccupations, the outlines of a pattern appeared, which I tried to focus on early on and repeated it in various interview situations whenever possible:

The fact that the patient, unconsciously, had such a fear of the loss of love and safety that she tended to avoid every conflict and argument, and was thus permanently under tension and suppressed anger, which were not communicated and therefore unresolved, but on the other hand, burdened the relationship even more than before, as opposed to the original intention of the defensive behavior. In addition, the patient felt the responsibility for this problem and for conflicts in the relationship.

From her past life, which I relate because it seemed so extremely vivid and present (actualized), as we often see in people with psychic problems, I will mention that the patient was an only child and felt lost between her powerless and devalued father and her dominating, imperious mother, who had a lover. Her mother pursued a divorce from her wrecked marriage, which led, after a horrible 10 years, to the loss of the mother. The patient was brought up by her grandmother and for a long time had an inconsolable and painful yearning for her mother.

In addition, her suppressed, undiagnosed myopia, as well as the connected weaknesses and deficiencies, had led to frequent criticisms and a feeling that as a child and as a girl she was not able to do anything right. Anxiety went with her obviously vivid temperament, and so she felt unloved, rejected, and surplus to requirement, and felt herself to be responsible for this and also the reason for her parents' quarrels, as well as, finally, their separation (no comment now on possible "oedipal" fantasies and guilt). Her own evil (bad girl) and guilt, which now in the session was accepted with hesitation, and which really was a new and amazing insight, not so much with respect to childhood but to her current relationship with her husband (mother).

In her first marriage to an alcoholic, who had been very dependent on her, and by whom she had been pregnant, she had obviously found a partner who helped her to manage her feelings of abandonment by not being the dependent one but rather the dominating partner. But bringing up her son alone in a marriage to an alcoholic was a disaster. She succeeded in growing, in mastering the situation as a mother, in her profession (secretary), and in life she found joy and reassurance by having more courage for activity. However, this was also (strenuous) and stressing, and her deep wish to be taken care for, to be sheltered, to have the passive feeling of being loved and adopted, were in no way fulfilled.

The activities of life, which were so important to her, made her independent and autonomous against old anxieties too, and she did many good things, which helped her to compensate, to balance guilty feelings coming up from frustration, disappointment, and rage.

At the time of this first marriage she met a man who became her lover. He was the opposite of the husband: a dominating, active man, a colleague in the same professional field, with whom she lived for many years in a dependent love–friendship–relationship, accompanied by increasing depression.

She loved him and could finally marry him, after (1) her son became an adult, and (2) after her (future) aged step-parents died one after the other, after sickness and being nursed by my patient! And after the husband had also broken off his former relationship to a woman with whom he had a daughter. What conditions for a marriage!

On the outside, good conditions finally, when it came to the fulfillment of wishes, but at that time complaints and symptoms became actualized and severe and the patient had to see her doctor increasingly often.

These facts were reconstructed during the course of two sessions, mainly asking ourselves why she was so defensive against aggression, and so full of tension.

Thus, there were some childhood and adult conditions, such as dependency and fear of loss, extramarital relationships, divorce, separation, care for difficult (step) parents, insecurity in marital relations, etc., that obviously played a major role in her adult life at that time.

But the patient did not challenge those problems with initiative, independence, and self-consciousness, certain demands, etc., she complained and suffered passive-dependently, and was angry about her background; therefore, she accused herself regarding her distrust (jealousy), instead of clearing up, finding solutions for her and her partner that she could live with. Why not?

The husband refused to become involved in long arguments meaning that they did not discuss things properly in the relationship.

He treated her lovingly on the face of it and for her perception, but a many things and discussions were forbidden, for her, not taking it seriously.

She only had a good life with regard to in housework and the garden, with no professional work, whereas over the past few years she had a great deal of pleasure, contacts, appreciation, and acceptance.

What became more clear to the patient during the course of two sessions (and I hope for you too) was that she got ill, because she could not solve an important actual (not conscious) problem by "modern," adult means, but rather in an anxiety-bound, regressive way or approach only, the problem and the immature solution both resembling an old problem and solution (transference):

Her old (neurotic) addiction of being dependent on affection and love, created from her fear of being left alone, inhibited her initiatives and her potential to argue, to quarrel in an adequate way, at least not without immediately feeling guilty about being bad and evil, and to have the responsibility for the difficulties in a relationship.

Her sensitivity regarding the dominating and imperious attitude of the husband, whom she loved and was sometimes jealous of and angry with at the same time, corresponded exactly to the sensitivity she had toward her mother, in childhood, with good reason. She did not want to risk the relationship and being abandoned, and for a really good relationship, of course, she risked much too little!

In addition, she came into conflict with her own success, with the position she had reached and her satisfaction and attractivity as a woman and as a professional by her own activities and initiatives.

With these interpretations, she realized that in the here-and-now reality she was probably less destructive in her activities and aggression, but more destructive in her inhibitions and defensive dissatisfaction, to which she felt forced by guilty feelings and fear of loss.

In her relationship with me there were similar (transferred) situations with this anxiety pattern: for example, when she did not understand immediately what I wanted to describe, and she denied this and tried to adapt, we then had a little misunderstanding, which led again to submission and adaption, and self-complaints about how stupid she was sometimes (with a little coquettish, flirtatious undertone … when she didn't feel too bad …).

Those little examples in the here-and-now situation may be most interesting, especially when we understand the "bothersome" feeling in the situation, obviously corresponding to the patient's message in her behavior: either you get angry, or you get seduced by submission (how good you are as a powerful object for the patient, or you want to help the depressed little girl, or you do not like addicted children who tend to panic, etc.). These may be feelings of countertransference, corresponding to the patient's unconscious or subliminal communication on various levels. They may lead us to ideas about the feeling and conflicts of the transferred relationship, and you can then clarify and interpret it with even more plausibility for the patient, because this is real and perceived and felt in the moment, and not only in the past or in the outside world with her husband. And it helps the patient to see herself from the outside.

After the second session, we had an interval of several weeks. She was increasingly relieved of her depression and suicidal thoughts, and, as I learned little by little from her in the subsequent third and fourth sessions, she had drawn the following conclusions (by her own direction, without any direct influence from me!):

- She tried to find some work and promptly found temporary but immediate work in a position in her old field as an appreciated colleague, even more than she could have wished for at the beginning.
- She talked to her husband and argued with him about different attitudes toward life, which diminished jealousy and distrust, with relief for the husband too.
- She was surprised that despite more tension in their arguments and in more aggressivity toward her husband, their relationship improved.

However, it turned out that he was not willing to cooperate more in changing for a better performance in the marriage, e.g., with the help of a couples session. But this no longer disturbed the patient as before (depression, anxiety).

In the fourth session, she felt no symptoms, and we discussed her only concerns, about what she could do in the case of a relapse to her former feelings and behavior.

Even if this does not seem like an everyday "quick cure," and even if there is a suspicion that adaption and positive feelings and identification with me play a role in this "quick cure," I think that the main idea can be shown and seen to be proven: that, within a valid method, focusing on a specific psychodynamic theme helps.

We cannot expect basic structural changes in behavior and personal disorders with short-term therapy or short consultations and interventions of this type (or, comparable in Balint work), but we can change something specific: as in this case, we can free the vitality and sthenicity, which were suppressed and went into a pathological alliance with pathogenic defense mechanisms, leading to autoaggressive symptoms, and by this induce a self-change, which the patient usually basically wishes for, despite all the chronic defensive behavior and habits and even secondary gratification by illness. With the help of a good enough relationship in therapy, and insight into the patient's anxieties, combined with their behavioral patterns in relationships, the patient gets the courage to venture in new directions.

We can show the patient their behavior in conflictual spaces, unconscious but close to their experience, and try to work this through using examples, with the small and large consequences and vicious circles.

The condition is that we can find out with the patient (not for the patient like objective data about their pathogenesis, "mentalization") a repeated subliminal conflictual field in their behavior, in their relationships with others and with themselves, that the patient can see and feel this more clearly and consciously when it is "mentalized," and perhaps understand it a little bit more from their past and the current life situation. All this is a basis for change in the patient's current life, which consists of helping and even challenging them not to retire from life, but to meet it again.

Chapter 4
Treatment of Major Depression in a Partial Hospital Program

Felicia Jackson, Melanie A. Hom, Elizabeth J. Lewis, and Thröstur Björgvinsson

Contents

F. Jackson
Department of Psychology, McLean Hospital, Belmont, MA, USA

Department of Psychiatry, Harvard Medical School, Boston, MA, USA

Jackson Psychological Services, Atlanta, GA, USA
e-mail: feliciajackson@jacksonpsych.com

M. A. Hom · E. J. Lewis · T. Björgvinsson (✉)
Department of Psychology, McLean Hospital, Belmont, MA, USA

Department of Psychiatry, Harvard Medical School, Boston, MA, USA
e-mail: mhom@mclean.harvard.edu; elewis@mclean.harvard.edu;
tbjorgvinsson@mclean.harvard.edu

© Springer Nature Switzerland AG 2021
C. Charis, G. Panayiotou (eds.), *Depression Conceptualization and Treatment*,
https://doi.org/10.1007/978-3-030-68932-2_4

4.1   Treatment of Major Depressive Disorder in Partial Settings

Major depressive disorder is among the most common psychiatric disorders globally and is a leading cause of impaired functioning and psychiatric hospitalization (Lépine & Briley, 2011). One setting to which individuals with major depressive disorder may present for treatment is a partial hospital program (PHP), which provides a bridge between inpatient and outpatient treatment. Although PHPs typically offer short-term treatment to an acute, high-risk patient population, they represent a surprisingly feasible and effective environment in which depression symptoms can be therapeutically impacted.

In this chapter, we will discuss how basic components of evidence-based treatment for depression can be seamlessly incorporated into a PHP to facilitate significant treatment gains and reductions in depression symptom severity in a short-term treatment model. We will briefly review gold-standard depression treatment approaches—largely informed by cognitive behavioral therapy (CBT) principles—and detail how these treatments can be administered in a PHP setting, drawing on our experiences at McLean Hospital's Behavioral Health Partial Hospital Program (BHP) in the United States (US). Through case vignettes, as well as a review of research and data from our own PHP, we will explore the important role of PHPs in patient care. We will additionally present ways PHPs not only provide vital clinical treatment but also can be designed to integrate research and clinical training to advance the mental health field.

4.2   Partial Hospital Programs as a "Bridge" in Treatment

For years, clinicians and researchers have observed a troubling trend in mental health treatment— the "revolving door" of psychiatric inpatient hospitalizations. This phenomenon is characterized by the frequent readmission of patients who were discharged to outpatient services from inpatient care, only to experience relapse and eventual return to inpatient hospitalization. Consider, for example, the experience of a severely depressed individual stuck in this revolving door. This individual, who is struggling with an acute mental health crisis, is first transitioned to an inpatient psychiatric hospital, where they spend several days on a locked unit. While on this unit, the patient is removed from real-life daily stressors, triggers, and responsibilities. They are also under near-constant observation, with high levels of support and precautions in place to limit harmful behaviors. During this hospitalization, treatment focuses primarily on stabilization, reduction of acute symptoms, and mitigating safety risks to clear thresholds for discharge. When the crisis subsides and the acute symptoms (e.g., mania, psychosis) stabilize, the patient is discharged to outpatient treatment.

Although this individual is likely returning to outpatient care with improved symptoms, they are immediately reentering their lives with substantially less support and often are no better equipped to handle their symptoms or stressors than they were prior to hospitalization. Through no fault of their own, the patient is left navigating a system with only two options: inpatient hospitalization or outpatient care. In this limited system, patients must make *too large of a step* from hospitalization to outpatient treatment. It follows, then, that patients may find themselves in a troubling back and forth between inpatient and outpatient care. This "revolving door" is burdensome not only for patients but also for the system. Indeed, in the year following discharge from inpatient hospitalization, over 50% of patients with major depressive disorder will be readmitted to inpatient care due to relapse or a worsening of symptoms (Lin et al., 2010; Shaffer et al., 2015). Beyond straining hospital systems, rehospitalizations can be significantly disruptive events in the lives of patients and their families (Mortensen & Eaton, 1994) and are often viewed as a sign of failure by patients, families, and providers (Lin et al., 2010). Being stuck in this revolving door can be taxing and understandably discouraging for all involved.

It is here where PHPs are useful; PHPs often serve as a bridge between inpatient and outpatient care. They provide a transition step that both (1) prioritizes the further stabilization of symptoms through intensive psychiatric care and (2) offers opportunities to learn skills to manage one's symptoms while being immersed in one's real life (e.g., living at home). In PHPs, patients learn new skills daily and can immediately practice those skills in real-life situations. Within 24 h, patients can review how they coped with these situations with their clinical team, discuss successes and struggles, and make adjustments guided by a clinician. In short, the goal of the PHP is to equip patients with skills to return to a level of functioning necessary to effectively engage in and fully benefit from outpatient treatment.

The US Code of Federal Regulations defines a PHP as "a time-limited, ambulatory, active treatment program that offers therapeutically intensive, coordinated, and structured clinical services within a stable therapeutic milieu" (United States (US) Government Publishing Office, 2018). PHPs are designed to provide care in lieu of inpatient hospitalization both to patients who are (1) "stepped up" from outpatient care due to the worsening of symptoms to avoid a crisis and inpatient hospitalization and (2) "stepped down" from hospitalization to further stabilize symptoms and prevent relapse (Leung, Drozd, & Maier, 2009). To be eligible for a PHP, patients cannot be at imminent risk of harming themselves or others; however, they are often at high risk for a worsening or relapse of acute symptoms, and they often present with nonzero risk to themselves and/or others (e.g., suicidal ideation without current intent or a plan; Björgvinsson et al., 2014).

Supporting the PHP as a model of care, research suggests that successfully connecting patients struggling with severe mental illness to community-based resources and/or behavioral health treatment reduces rehospitalization and can improve quality of life (Ilgen, Hu, Moos, & McKellar, 2008; Nelson, Maruish, & Axler, 2000). Even when these transition-focused interventions are brief (e.g., the brief critical time intervention; Shaffer et al., 2015), they can reduce rehospitalizations both over the short and long term and, thus, serving as an invaluable point along the care continuum.

4.3   Structure and Function of a Partial Hospital Program

PHPs provide intensive day treatment in a highly structured environment. In general, PHP patients' daily schedules involve multiple treatment modalities (e.g., group and individual therapy), case management, and consultation with psychopharmacologists and other providers (e.g., vocational counselors, occupational therapists; International Commission on Accreditation of Rehabilitation Facilities, 2016). A PHP treatment team is often composed of a multidisciplinary team of mental health providers, including psychiatrists, clinical psychologists, social workers, mental health counselors, community residence counselors, and trainees.

The Behavioral Health Partial Hospital Program (BHP) at McLean Hospital can be used as an illustrative example of a PHP. With over 850 admissions each year, the BHP provides intensive treatment for adults (i.e., individuals aged 18 years and older) experiencing acute psychopathology (e.g., mood and anxiety disorders, personality psychopathology, mania, psychosis, and substance use problems).

Patients attend the program Monday through Friday, from 8:30 am to 3:00 pm, and are enrolled on average for eight program days. Patients first report to the program building, sign in, and complete a daily self-assessment questionnaire to monitor symptoms and track progress (discussed in greater detail below). Starting at 9:00 am, patients attend a 50-min group session every hour (with the exception of the 12:00 pm hour), totaling up to five groups each day. Multiple groups are offered every hour, with approximately 80 unique evidence-based, protocol-driven groups offered weekly. The number of patients attending each group range from 2 to 15, with group sizes varying largely due to the subject matter and focus of the group. For example, foundational CBT skills groups typically include a large number of patients, while groups on psychotic symptoms or personality disorders are smaller and more focused on content. On average, 28 patients attend the program each day, with over 850 admissions per year (approximately 70 per month).

The BHP clinical team consists of clinical psychologists, psychology trainees (i.e., practicum students, doctoral interns, and postdoctoral fellows), social workers, psychiatrists, nurses, and bachelor's level counselors. Upon admission to the program, each patient is assigned an individual clinical team manager (CTM), psychiatrist, and program therapist, with whom the patient meets two to three times each week for 15- to 30-min sessions. The BHP milieu also includes a research team—composed of staff psychologists, postdoctoral fellows, a research coordinator, and research assistants—all of whom play an integral role in data collection and progress monitoring efforts.

A CTM provides case management; they complete an initial intake assessment, coordinate PHP services, and oversee aftercare planning. Group and individual skills-based therapy are provided by clinical psychologists, psychology trainees, and counselors. A psychiatrist provides psychopharmacology consultation, and other appointments are scheduled and provided as needed (e.g., vocational counseling, family meetings).

Through group and individual therapy, patients learn and practice skills from evidence-based treatments, including CBT (Beck, 2011), dialectical behavior therapy (DBT; Linehan, 2015), and acceptance and commitment therapy (ACT; Hayes, Strosahl, & Wilson, 2012). Patients also participate in process groups (e.g., support groups for those living with mood and anxiety disorders), self-assessment groups (e.g., CBT diary card, chain analysis), and general skills groups (e.g., communication skills, crisis planning, and coping with loss). Individualized group schedules are created by the CTM after initial assessment and are adjusted as needed throughout treatment. Patients are assigned to groups that best fit their needs; for example, patients presenting with severe depression will likely be assigned to several behavioral activation groups, a psychoeducation group about depression, and a process support group for those living with mood and anxiety disorders and other general skills training groups.

A unique and critical component of PHP care is that, at the end of each day, patients return home and to their daily lives. This program design comes with some costs. For instance, returning home in the late afternoon each day means that patients—especially those who are severely depressed or high risk—have fewer behavioral limitations. Patients thus have the chance to engage in any number of risky, dangerous, or impulsive behaviors such as self-injury, substance use, or interpersonal conflicts. Efforts to mitigate these risks are described in detail in our case vignettes and include safety planning, regular check-ins with the treatment team, progress monitoring to track increases in symptoms, and frequent communication between the treatment team and clinical staff who have observed changes in patient presentation throughout the day. At the same time, this model comes with significant benefits. Going home each afternoon allows patients to practice returning to their lives while learning new skills and receiving extensive support from their treatment team. Engaging in real-world skills application, while still receiving intensive support, decreases the likelihood of risky behaviors.

As an aside, at the time of our writing this chapter, we have also begun exploring alternate PHP delivery approaches. Prompted by the shift to virtual care that occurred in response to the COVID-19 pandemic, we developed an entirely virtual version of our PHP. By leveraging a secure web-based videoconferencing platform and other collaborative workspace platforms, our staff has been able to continue providing intensive psychiatric services to acute psychiatric patients (see Hom et al., 2020, for details regarding our transition to virtual care delivery). Thus far, treatment outcomes and patient satisfaction appear to be comparable to that in our in-person PHP, perhaps, in part, because patient participation from home facilitates improved practice of skills within one's home context. We note this virtual effort to emphasize that there may be many viable avenues and formats by which to deliver PHP-level care.

4.4   Cognitive Behavioral Therapy for Depression and the Role of Behavioral Activation (BA)

CBT is the gold-standard treatment approach for major depressive disorder. Supported by an extensive literature spanning decades (see Butler, Chapman, Forman, & Beck, 2006, for meta-analytic review), the basic CBT model of depression suggests that distorted negative thoughts and beliefs (e.g., about the self, others, and/or the world), paired with maladaptive behavioral patterns (e.g., a lack of involvement in pleasant activities, social isolation, difficulties functioning at work and school), lead to the development and maintenance of depressed mood. Depressed mood and anhedonia then foster additional unhelpful behaviors and negative belief patterns, further driving functional impairments. Given this model, CBT for depression targets maladaptive thinking patterns and unhelpful behaviors to improve mood (Beck, 2011). As stated previously, CBT is the primary treatment model utilized at the BHP; in particular, there is a focus on leveraging BA principles.

Nearly 45 years ago, Lewinsohn, Biglan, and Zeiss (1976) introduced their seminal work on the behavioral treatment of major depression. Rooted in the principle that depression is characterized by a lack of engagement in positively reinforcing or meaningful activities due to anhedonia, lack of motivation, and the general fatigue associated with depressive episodes, they proposed that depression symptoms could be effectively reduced by facilitating engagement in pleasurable activities and re-engaging with meaningful, positive activities. Since that time, the field has amassed expansive literature supporting both the efficacy and effectiveness of *behavioral activation* in the treatment of depression (see Mazzucchelli, Kane, & Rees, 2009, for meta-analytic review). Some research has also suggested that the greatest therapeutic gains in CBT for depression are achieved in early sessions when BA is administered (Cullen, Spates, Pagoto, & Doran, 2006).

The concept of sudden gains early in treatment may be a core element of change in the PHP setting—given our BHP's brief, high-intensity approach to treatment, from Day 1, patients are thrust into a world largely consistent with concepts of behavioral activation. Built into the PHP model are daily structure, socialization, and support, all of which are explicit goals of BA. Indeed, research from our BHP suggests that BA is a critical component in treating depression at this level of care (Webb, Kertz, Bigda-Peyton, & Björgvinsson, 2013). At admission, our patients are often struggling with social isolation, lack of daily structure, poor sleep, poor self-care, and limited engagement in pleasant activities. The strict daily structure and social component of the BHP allow multiple BA interventions to occur simultaneously. For example, the program requires that patients arrive by 8:30 am each day and attend group sessions every hour. Over a typical 10-day stay, the structure of the PHP serves as an intervention for dysregulated sleep. Sleep hygiene is also a topic of group and individual sessions, which aids in eliminating harmful sleep habits. Further, from the start, patients are immersed in a community of 20–30 "fellow travelers"—their peers in the program. In addition to having frequent social interactions with peers in therapy groups, during lunch, and between sessions, patients may also benefit from peer validation, encouragement, and reminders that they are not alone in their struggles. This program milieu allows patients to feel like they are part of a community and directly leverages BA principles.

Of note, our PHP does not rely entirely on traditional CBT and BA for the treatment of depression. As previously noted, BHP patients receive group and individual instruction on third-wave approaches including DBT and ACT, which may scaffold the CBT and BA interventions and further fuel symptom reduction. For instance, a depressed patient might be assigned to attend an ACT-based group on values and committed action. In this group, the patient learns to identify values and explores how values can increase willingness to engage in values-driven actions (Wilson & Murrell, 2004). Patients then complete a worksheet in session, setting concrete goals for values-driven action, explicitly stating how anchoring to their values can increase their willingness to complete their goals. In this way, exercises that integrate ACT-based principles may increase a patient's likelihood of following through with BA plans and further support treatment goals.

DBT skills also bolster depressed patients' ability to make behavioral changes. For example, a depressed patient may attend a DBT group discussing emotion regulation and the importance of (1) accumulating positive emotions through pleasurable activities and (2) engaging in activities that build mastery to decrease vulnerability to negative emotions (Linehan, 2015). DBT groups introducing interpersonal effectiveness skills may help patients practice communicating their needs, therefore increasing rewarding interpersonal interactions—a particularly important skill in the treatment of severe, chronic depression (McCullough, 2003). Distress tolerance groups foster the development of skills for tolerating emotional crises; a patient may learn to practice deep breathing or to "TIPP" their body temperature using cold water in order to navigate difficult situations without engaging in risky behaviors.

In sum, this integrative approach to the treatment of depression that can be provided in a PHP setting allows patients to benefit not only from active psychoeducation and multifaceted treatment approaches but also from the daily structure, social milieu, skills training, and ability to practice these new skills in real time in their home context. We believe the combination of these elements may contribute to the observed sudden gains in functioning and reductions in depression observed among our patients from pre- to posttreatment (Björgvinsson et al., 2014).

To illustrate this process, in the sections that follow, we will demonstrate through case examples how the PHP structure, combined with the integration of CBT and third-wave therapeutic techniques and skills training, can be effective in the treatment of a high-risk patient population with severe depression symptoms, multiple psychiatric comorbidities, and elevated suicide risk. Further, we will review ways in which a PHP creates a surprisingly ideal environment that allows for the integration of clinical research and training, completing an institution-wide tripartite mission of research, training, and treatment.

4.5   Case Vignette #1: Treatment of a Patient with Multiple Comorbidities

"Jesse" was a 20-year-old transgender male presenting to the BHP with worsening depression, anxiety, marijuana use, and posttraumatic stress symptoms—in addition to increased suicidal ideation and borderline personality traits—in the context of work and social stressors. Jesse had a difficult childhood with multiple traumas, an extensive history of self-harm, and several suicide attempts; he had previously received treatment for borderline personality disorder. He struggled with issues of gender dysphoria and shame surrounding wanting to transition to male while growing up in a conservative household. Jesse reported that many of his depression symptoms decreased once he began transitioning, stating that he finally started to feel like himself. He went to college and found his "chosen family" in deep relationships at school and work. However, a perfect storm of a romantic breakup following a sexual assault within that relationship and discrimination at work for being transgender sent him back into the depths of suicidality and depression. Jesse presented to the BHP at the referral of his outpatient therapist to learn additional skills and for an assessment of additional treatment options.

Jesse began the intake session stating that he was not sure this program would be helpful to him, as the skills seemed very general and he had already completed DBT. His treatment team assured him that they work hard to tailor treatment to him and to assess where the missing links in his skills use were that were resulting in his engaging in harmful behaviors (e.g., cutting, gathering means for suicide, substance use, risky sexual behavior). Although Jesse met the criteria for multiple psychiatric disorders per the Mini-International Neuropsychiatric Interview (MINI; Sheehan et al., 1998), he identified that the symptoms most distressing to him were depressed mood and flashback-related panic-associated symptoms that led to engagement in the aforementioned problem behaviors.

His individual sessions began with a comprehensive safety plan that included identifying his (1) triggers for self-harm and gathering means for suicide, (2) internal coping strategies (e.g., updating his DBT distress tolerance kit), (3) external coping strategies (e.g., identifying people to call for distraction and support), (4) his treaters, (5) the location of his local emergency room, (6) ideas for making his environment safe, and (7) a reminder of his values and reasons for living. To his surprise, Jesse found groups to be helpful, enjoying the mix of CBT, DBT, and ACT skills. Jesse was eager to address his posttraumatic stress symptoms but was encouraged to first master distress tolerance skills to prepare for future outpatient trauma treatment. He refined his distress tolerance skills to more effectively ride out self-harm and substance use urges (e.g., by taking long walks while listening to soothing music). The treatment fell over a holiday, which the patient was spending alone for the first time in his life, and he was able to schedule and complete a detailed plan for the day that included spending time with friends earlier in the evening without using substances and engaging in valued self-care activities, such as crocheting.

Jesse encountered several stressors during BHP treatment, including a panic attack following a sexual experience that turned nonconsensual. He felt he was able to ride the panic attack out without engaging in problem behaviors due to the use of various distress tolerance skills (e.g., tipping his body temperature with cold water; Linehan, 2015). With increased control over his behavior, the patient felt confident enough to leave the program with additional referrals to a DBT for posttraumatic stress disorder outpatient program and a support group for college students experiencing mental health issues. His BHP CTM ran into him in the halls several times post-discharge when the patient was on his way to these meetings, and each time, the patient reported his life was slowly and surely beginning to look up.

4.6 Case Vignette #2: Risk Assessment and Management

Given the clinical severity of our patient population, it is not uncommon for safety and risk management concerns to arise. Consider the case of Anna, a 21-year-old single bisexual cisgender female who presented to the PHP as a step-up from outpatient care due to worsening depression and suicidal ideation. At admission, Anna reported to her CTM and psychiatrist that she had been experiencing suicidal ideation daily and was considering overdosing on medications. She reported two psychiatric hospitalizations in the past year, both following suicide attempts with a high degree of potential lethality. Anna also reported frequent thoughts of hurting herself on the Patient Health Questionnaire-9 (PHQ-9; Kroenke, Spitzer, & Williams, 2001) at admission, and she reported active suicidal ideation with some intent but no specific plans during a structured interview (i.e., the Columbia-Suicide Severity Rating Scale [C-SSRS]; Posner et al., 2011) with her program therapist. Integrating these and other clinical data, at admission, her treatment team considered her to be at elevated but not imminent suicide risk (Chu et al., 2015). Additionally, because Anna expressed a high degree of motivation to engage in PHP treatment, the BHP was determined to be an appropriate level of care for her.

To manage risk, on Anna's first day in the program, she and her CTM worked together to create a personalized safety plan, and she agreed to restrict her access to her medications (Stanley & Brown, 2012). During Anna's time at the BHP, her treatment team frequently communicated about her risk and clinical status via email and phone, during team rounds, and in-person, as needed. Her BHP team ensured that Anna was scheduled to see at least two providers for individual sessions each day to facilitate increased clinical contact and opportunities for risk assessment. Clinical information captured by her PHP treatment team was supplemented by Anna's daily progress monitoring data and behavioral observations from other PHP staff based on her engagement in group sessions and interactions with peers in the milieu. Over the course of her 10-day stay, Anna reported—both in individual sessions with her PHP treatment team and on her daily progress monitoring forms—steady improvement in her depression symptoms and a reduction in the severity and intensity of her suicidal thoughts. After a family meeting with her parents to discuss her aftercare plans, Anna was discharged to her outpatient treatment team.

This vignette highlights numerous features of the BHP that allow for the effective, timely management of risk and safety concerns among patients presenting with depression. For one, we have the opportunity to integrate clinical data from multiple sources to inform our assessment and management of risk (e.g., self-report and clinical interview data, behavioral observations). These data are collected daily and across multiple settings (e.g., group and individual sessions, the milieu). Our approach to risk assessment and management is also empirically informed; we use validated measures (e.g., PHQ-9, C-SSRS) and interventions with a robust evidence base (e.g., safety planning; Stanley & Brown, 2012). This vignette also demonstrates our PHP's capacity to adapt care based on patients' unique needs—in the case of Anna, ensuring multiple individual meetings with providers daily. Finally, this example illustrates the value the BHP places on open and frequent communication between members of the treatment team, which is key to effective risk management. Of note, if at any point Anna's team had determined that she was at imminent suicide risk, they would have pursued a more intensive level of care for her. Because the BHP is situated within a hospital that provides comprehensive psychiatric services, CTMs can seamlessly oversee the direct hand-off of BHP patients to inpatient hospital staff, often with a recommendation for patients to return to the BHP after crisis stabilization.

4.7   The Role of Clinical Assessment and Research

Ongoing assessment is central to the delivery of CBT for depression; it informs case conceptualization, treatment planning, and modifications to treatment approach (Dobson & Dobson, 2017). At our PHP, clinical data are routinely and systematically collected through daily progress monitoring surveys and structured clinical interviews.

For daily progress monitoring, patients complete a self-report survey battery on a secure web-based platform each morning before PHP programming begins. The battery is composed of validated measures that assess a range of domains relevant to PHP care, including multiple depression symptom indices (e.g., the Patient Health Questionnaire-9 [Kroenke et al., 2001]). Reports summarizing each patient's responses are generated automatically and uploaded daily for each clinical team to review. Reports include total scores and item-level responses for measures, graphical depictions of day-to-day changes in symptom measure scores since admission, and indicators of whether patients are reporting clinically significant symptoms based on established cutoffs. A patient's clinical team is also alerted via email if they report a concerning change in symptoms (e.g., more frequent suicidal thoughts).

In this context, progress monitoring serves multiple functions. These data inform a team's initial assessment (e.g., diagnostics, risk determinations) and treatment planning (e.g., group schedule). Trends over time also signal whether the program is yielding therapeutic benefits or whether a patient may benefit from alternate or more intensive levels of care. Further, these data can guide aftercare plans—for instance, by revealing if a patient with depression might benefit from a substance use treatment program. Finally, *how* the patients complete the surveys is clinically useful. For example, unusually long survey completion times, difficulties understanding questions, or consistent denial of any psychiatric symptoms can all be informative.

In addition to daily progress monitoring, PHP patients complete a structured clinical interview with their program therapist on their second day of treatment. This interview is composed of measures assessing (1) whether a patient meets diagnostic criteria for a range of psychiatric disorders, (2) a patient's history of suicidality and non-suicidal self-injury, (3) functional impairments associated with a patient's psychiatric problems, and (4) a patient's overall symptom severity. Program therapists report findings from this interview to other clinical team members. As with the progress monitoring data, interview results inform treatment planning and aftercare selection. This interview is especially useful in guiding case conceptualization and diagnostics; its structured format aids differential diagnosis and can reveal concerns not readily apparent at admission (e.g., social anxiety secondary to primary depression).

Progress monitoring and clinical interview data not only guide patient care at the individual level but also are routinely aggregated to evaluate program-level treatment outcomes, including depression outcomes. At discharge, patients are also asked to provide feedback regarding their treatment experiences. This feedback is then used to shape ongoing programmatic improvement efforts. At this juncture, it is worth briefly noting that the BHP has an active research arm (see Forgeard, Beard, Kirakosian, & Björgvinsson, 2018, for a detailed description). Indeed, the BHP and our overarching institution are committed to advancing scientific discovery. All patients can consent for their de-identified progress monitoring and clinical interview data, as well as data from their medical charts, to be used in research. Moreover, ancillary studies are often conducted at our PHP, which patients can opt to participate in, if interested. Critically, research is viewed by our staff as having the potential to improve the services we provide, and PHP-based research projects are thoughtfully designed to minimize burden on patients—both factors have been key in facilitating the relatively seamless integration of research into our clinical program.

4.8   Depression Treatment Outcomes in the Partial Hospital Program Setting

As illustrated in the case vignettes, the collection of clinical data at the BHP also allows for the measurement of treatment outcomes. Utilizing the Clinical Global Impressions Scale-Severity (CGI-S; Guy, 1976), program therapists use their clinical observations and judgment to rate patients' current symptom severity at admission on a 7-point Likert-type scale from 1 ("Minimal") to 7 ("Extremely Severe"). At admission, approximately 75% of depressed patients presenting to our PHP are rated from 5 ("Marked") to 7 ("Extremely Severe") at admission. However, by the discharge, only 30% of these patients are rated 5 ("Marked") or higher. Moreover, on the CGI-Improvement (CGI-I; Guy, 1976), 46% of our depressed patients were rated by clinicians as "Very much" or "Much" improved at discharge, and 85% of depressed patients were observed to be at least "Minimally" improved at discharge.

In addition to clinician indices of treatment progress, patients also completed self-report measures that capture daily symptom changes and changes from admission to discharge. These include both depression symptom measures (e.g., the PHQ-9; Kroenke et al., 2001) and measures of symptoms commonly associated with depression (e.g., the Generalized Anxiety Disorder Screener; Spitzer, Kroenke, Williams, & Löwe, 2006). Together, these measures allow us to assess individual- and program-level treatment outcomes. Based on these data, we have found that 60% of BHP patients present with a diagnosis of a current major depressive episode, as assessed by the MINI (Sheehan et al., 1998). On the C-SSRS (Posner et al., 2011), 47% of patients report moderate to severe suicidal ideation, and approximately 20% report having engaged in suicidal behaviors in the past month. From admission to discharge, patients, on average, appear to report a significant and clinically meaningful reduction in depression symptom severity, with 30% of patients reporting recovery from depression based on self-report measures (Björgvinsson et al., 2014).

4.9 Integration of Training and Supervision in a Partial Hospital Setting

One might suspect that the integration of training and supervision in a PHP setting would be challenging. Although there are many moving parts, the PHP environment creates many opportunities for rich training experiences with patients with acute psychopathology in a setting in which many licensed clinicians are available for trainees should crises arise.

In any given year, McLean's BHP is the home site for six to eight doctoral students to complete their predoctoral clinical internship—the capstone applied experience of the clinical psychology doctoral degree in the United States. Research and clinical work are inherently integrated at the BHP, allowing interns with a range of interests to meet their training goals during this primarily clinically focused year. The BHP additionally recruits three to six advanced graduate students (i.e., practicum students) from local, national, and occasionally international doctoral programs. Both doctoral interns and practicum students serve as group co-leaders and individual program therapists. The BHP also typically has two postdoctoral fellows, one who is more clinically focused (e.g., co-directs the practicum program) and the other who is more research-focused (e.g., supervises assessment-related training). Both fellows often serve as group co-facilitators and program therapists.

Each trainee receives supervision in various formats, all of which are designed to help the trainee feel safe in developing their clinical decision-making skills and empowered to grow into an independent clinician. Each trainee is assigned two to four supervisors with whom they meet weekly one-on-one to discuss clinical and professional issues. Trainees are encouraged to use supervision time to meet their training goals and needs (e.g., discussing different patients with each supervisor or discussing their most challenging patient with multiple supervisors to hear different conceptualizations of the patient's presenting problems and treatment options).

The trainee then acts as an independent consultant to the treatment team. Treatment teams meet weekly in group rounds to discuss and coordinate clinical care. The psychiatrist and CTM often weigh in on the trainee's work with the patient, but it is understood both that the trainee is consulting independent supervisors on these cases as well and that trainees are using their best judgment in their work with each patient. Trainees and CTMs communicate frequently off-line as well—after each program therapy session, the trainee leaves a voicemail "sign out" for the CTM so that the CTM can track the patient's progress and remain apprised of what skills the patient is finding most helpful to guide aftercare planning. Trainees also page CTMs when acute risk concerns arise (e.g., imminent suicide risk) to facilitate further risk assessment and safety planning. CTMs and psychiatrists additionally serve as ad hoc supervisors by guiding and providing feedback on trainees' risk assessment approaches and clinical decision-making.

Finally, that the BHP is a training program at its core creates an environment in which a growth mindset permeates, with routine training and seminars offered to the broader BHP staff (e.g., CTMs, psychiatrists, nurses, and counselors). The BHP's weekly staff meetings are a space for the dissemination of information, group discussion and decision-making, and staff-wide training (e.g., where diverse speakers are invited to share their knowledge on research or clinical topics). Therefore, while at first blush, it may appear that there would be complications to having a training program embedded within a PHP, in our experience, this model creates a vibrant training environment for all staff members, such that learning is reinforced on a daily basis. It is understood that this process of learning is never fully finished.

4.10 Conclusions

In this chapter, we have reviewed our approach to the evidence-based treatment of depression in a partial hospital program (PHP) setting. By discussing the format and structure of our PHP, presenting case vignettes, and discussing the integration of research and training into our treatment model, we illustrated the feasibility and promise of PHP-level care in treating depression and bolstering continuity of care among patients with severe psychopathology. Given the multifaceted, interdisciplinary approach to treatment in a PHP, efforts are needed to better understand the specific mechanisms of change that facilitate the sudden gains and depression symptom reductions we have observed at our own US-based PHP. We look forward to the adoption of similar models of care elsewhere and hope that other mental health treatment providers and systems might consider the benefits of this unique bridge between inpatient and outpatient psychiatric care.

Acknowledgment We would like to thank the staff and patients of the Behavioral Health Partial Hospital at McLean Hospital.

References

Beck, J. S. (2011). *Cognitive behavior therapy, Second Edition: Basics and beyond.* New York, NY: The Guilford Press.

Björgvinsson, T., Kertz, S. J., Bigda-Peyton, J. S., Rosmarin, D. H., Aderka, I. M., & Neuhaus, E. C. (2014). Effectiveness of cognitive behavior therapy for severe mood disorders in an acute psychiatric naturalistic setting: A benchmarking study. *Cognitive Behaviour Therapy, 43*(3), 209–220. https://doi.org/10.1080/16506073.2014.901988

Butler, A. C., Chapman, J. E., Forman, E. M., & Beck, A. T. (2006). The empirical status of cognitive-behavioral therapy: A review of meta-analyses. *Clinical Psychology Review, 26*(1), 17–31. https://doi.org/10.1016/j.cpr.2005.07.003

Chu, C., Klein, K. M., Buchman-Schmitt, J. M., Hom, M. A., Hagan, C. R., & Joiner, T. E. (2015). Routinized assessment of suicide risk in clinical practice: An empirically informed update. *Journal of Clinical Psychology, 71*(12), 1186–1200. https://doi.org/10.1002/jclp.22210

Cullen, J. M., Spates, C. R., Pagoto, S., & Doran, N. (2006). Behavioral activation treatment for major depressive disorder: A pilot investigation. *The Behavior Analyst Today, 7*(1), 151–166. https://doi.org/10.1037/h0100150

Dobson, D. J. G., & Dobson, K. S. (2017). *Evidence-based practice of cognitive-behavioral therapy* (2nd ed.). New York, NY: The Guilford Press.

Forgeard, M., Beard, C., Kirakosian, N., & Björgvinsson, T. (2018). Research in partial hospital settings. In *Practice-based research* (pp. 212–240). London: Routledge. https://doi.org/10.432 4/9781315524610-12

Guy, W. (1976). *ECDEU assessment manual for psychopharmacology.* Bethesda, MD: National Institute of Mental Health (NIMH), National Institutes of Health (NIH).

Hayes, S. C., Strosahl, K. D., & Wilson, K. G. (2012). *Acceptance and commitment therapy: The process and practice of mindful change* (2nd ed.). New York, NY: Guilford Press.

Hom, M. A., Weiss, R. B., Millman, Z. B., Christensen, K., Lewis, E. J., Cho, S., … Björgvinsson, T. (2020). Development of a virtual partial hospital program for an acute psychiatric population: Lessons learned and future directions for telepsychotherapy. *Journal of Psychotherapy Integration, 3*, 366. https://doi.org/10.1037/int0000212

Ilgen, M. A., Hu, K. U., Moos, R. H., & McKellar, J. (2008). Continuing care after inpatient psychiatric treatment for patients with psychiatric and substance use disorders. *Psychiatric Services, 59*(9), 982–988. https://doi.org/10.1176/ps.2008.59.9.982

International Commission on Accreditation of Rehabilitation Facilities (CARF). (2016). *Partial hospitalization.* Retrieved from http://www.carf.org/Programs/ProgramDescriptions/BH-Partial-Hospitalization/

Kroenke, K., Spitzer, R. L., & Williams, J. B. (2001). The PHQ-9: Validity of a brief depression severity measure. *Journal of General Internal Medicine, 16*(9), 606–613. https://doi.org/10.1046/j.1525-1497.2001.016009606.x

Lépine, J. P., & Briley, M. (2011). The increasing burden of depression. *Neuropsychiatric Disease and Treatment, 7*(Suppl), 3–7. https://doi.org/10.2147/NDT.S19617

Leung, M. Y., Drozd, E. M., & Maier, J. (2009). *Impact associated with the Medicare psychiatric PPS: A study of partial hospital programs.* Retrieved from https://www.cms.gov/Research-Statistics-Data-and-Systems/Statistics-Trends-and-Reports/Reports/downloads/Leung_PHP_PPS_2010.pdf

Lewinsohn, P. M., Biglan, A., & Zeiss, A. M. (1976). Behavioral treatment of depression. In P. O. Davidson (Ed.), *The behavioral management of anxiety, depression and pain* (pp. 91–146). New York, NY: Brunner/Mazel.

Lin, C. H., Chen, M. C., Chou, L. S., Lin, C. H., Chen, C. C., & Lane, H. Y. (2010). Time to rehospitalization in patients with major depression vs. those with schizophrenia or bipolar I disorder in a public psychiatric hospital. *Psychiatry Research, 180*(2–3), 74–79. https://doi.org/10.1016/j.psychres.2009.12.003

Linehan, M. M. (2015). *DBT® skills training manual* (2nd ed.). New York, NY: Guilford Press.

Mazzucchelli, T., Kane, R., & Rees, C. (2009). Behavioral activation treatments for depression in adults: A meta-analysis and review. *Clinical Psychology: Science and Practice, 16*(4), 383–411. https://doi.org/10.1111/j.1468-2850.2009.01178.x

McCullough, J. P. (2003). Treatment for chronic depression using Cognitive Behavioral Analysis System of Psychotherapy (CBASP). *Journal of Clinical Psychology, 59*(8), 833–846. https://doi.org/10.1002/jclp.10176

Mortensen, P. B., & Eaton, W. W. (1994). Predictors for readmission risk in schizophrenia. *Psychological Medicine, 24*(1), 223–232. https://doi.org/10.1017/S0033291700026982

Nelson, E. A., Maruish, M. E., & Axler, J. L. (2000). Effects of discharge planning and compliance with outpatient appointments on readmission rates. *Psychiatric Services, 51*(7), 885–889. https://doi.org/10.1176/appi.ps.51.7.885

Posner, K., Brown, G., Stanley, B., Brent, D., Yershova, K., Oquendo, M., … Mann, J. (2011). The Columbia-Suicide Severity Rating Scale: Initial validity and internal consistency findings from three multisite studies with adolescents and adults. *American Journal of Psychiatry, 168*(12), 1266–1277. https://doi.org/10.1176/appi.ajp.2011.10111704

Shaffer, S. L., Hutchison, S. L., Ayers, A. M., Goldberg, R. W., Herman, D., Duch, D. A., … Terhorst, L. (2015). Brief critical time intervention to reduce psychiatric rehospitalization. *Psychiatric Services, 66*(11), 1155–1161. https://doi.org/10.1176/appi.ps.201400362

Sheehan, D. V., Lecrubier, Y., Sheehan, K. H., Amorim, P., Janavs, J., Weiller, E., … Dunbar, G. C. (1998). The Mini-International Neuropsychiatric Interview (M.I.N.I.): The development and validation of a structured diagnostic psychiatric interview for DSM-IV and ICD-10. *Journal of Clinical Psychiatry, 59*(Suppl 20), 22–33.

Spitzer, R. L., Kroenke, K., Williams, J. B. W., & Löwe, B. (2006). A brief measure for assessing generalized anxiety disorder: The GAD-7. *Archives of Internal Medicine, 166*(10), 1092–1097. https://doi.org/10.1001/archinte.166.10.1092

Stanley, B., & Brown, G. K. (2012). Safety planning intervention: A brief intervention to mitigate suicide risk. *Cognitive and Behavioral Practice, 19*(2), 256–264. https://doi.org/10.1016/j.cbpra.2011.01.001

The Federal Government of the United States. (2018). *Title 32 code of federal regulations.* Washington, DC: United States (U.S.) Government Publishing Office.

Webb, C. A., Kertz, S. J., Bigda-Peyton, J. S., & Björgvinsson, T. (2013). The role of pretreatment outcome expectancies and cognitive-behavioral skills in symptom improvement in an acute psychiatric setting. *Journal of Affective Disorders, 149*(1–3), 375–382. https://doi.org/10.1016/j.jad.2013.02.016

Wilson, K. G., & Murrell, A. R. (2004). Values work in acceptance and commitment therapy: Setting a course for behavioral treatment. In S. C. Hayes, V. M. Follette, & M. M. Linehan (Eds.), *Mindfulness & acceptance: Expanding the cognitive-behavioral tradition* (pp. 120–151). New York, NY: Guilford Press.

Chapter 5
Psychodynamic Theory and Approaches to Depression

Fredric N. Busch

Contents

5.1 Introduction

Psychopharmacological treatments, interpersonal psychotherapy, and various forms of cognitive behavioral therapies for depressive disorders have predominated in the psychiatric and psychological literature in recent years. Although these approaches have demonstrated efficacy in randomized controlled trials (American Psychiatric Association, 2010; CANMAT, 2016), many patients do not respond fully to these treatments, demonstrating recurrent or persistent depression and ongoing problems in psychosocial functioning (Eaton, Shao, Nestadt, Lee, Bievnvenu, Zandi et al., 2008; Judd, Akiskal, & Paulus, 1997; Keller, Hanks, & Klein, 1996; Kocsis &

A note in the text is necessary to state that this chapter is drawn from chapters 1 and 2 of Busch, Rudden & Shapiro. Psychodynamic Treatment of Depression. American Psychiatric Press, second edition, 2016.

F. N. Busch (✉)
Columbia University Center for Psychoanalytic Training and Research, New York, NY, USA

Well Cornell Medical College, New York, NY, USA

© Springer Nature Switzerland AG 2021
C. Charis, G. Panayiotou (eds.), *Depression Conceptualization and Treatment*,
https://doi.org/10.1007/978-3-030-68932-2_5

Klein, 1995; Vieta, Sanchez-Moreno, Lahuerta, Zaragoza, EDHIPO group et al., 2008). Therefore, it is important to continue to develop and study treatments for depression.

Although used by a large number of clinicians, psychodynamic approaches to depression have not been researched as extensively, although evidence thus far suggests they are efficacious (Driessen et al., 2010; Leichsenring, Leweke, Klein, & Steinert, 2015). However, many of these studies employ traditional psychodynamic treatments that do not focus on specific disorders, instead broadly addressing the problems patients present with. The utility of psychodynamic treatments for specific disorders has been enhanced by using manualized approaches that focus on psychodynamic factors of these specific problems. My colleagues and I have been involved in the development of a series of such approaches for anxiety disorders (Busch, Milrod, Singer, & Aronson, 2012), depression (Busch, Rudden, & Shapiro, 2016), and posttraumatic stress disorder (Busch, Milrod, Chen & Singer, in press), as well as behavioral problems (Busch, 2018). One of these treatments, panic-focused psychodynamic psychotherapy, has demonstrated efficacy in randomized controlled trials for panic disorder (Busch et al., 2012, while the others have not been tested. A potential value of psychodynamic treatments is that addressing contributory dynamic factors may have a broader impact on vulnerability to persistence or recurrence of depression and psychosocial difficulties.

Theoreticians have developed a variety of models to explain why certain individuals develop depressive disorders and to develop effective interventions. Vulnerability to depression has been explained variously in terms of biochemical, interpersonal, psychodynamic, and cognitive-behavioral models. The psychodynamic approach provides an understanding and treatment of depression that is complementary to other models and approaches. In this chapter, I will provide a brief summary of psychoanalytic theories of depression, describe studies of psychological factors associated with this disorder, and present a psychodynamic formulation that can be employed in guiding treatment. A brief clinical example will illustrate how these approaches can be used in a given patient with depression.

5.2 Psychodynamic Models of Depression

Psychoanalysts have developed a series of models to understand and address the etiology and persistence of depressive syndromes. These models have considered the individual's biological and temperamental vulnerabilities, the quality of the person's earliest attachment relationships, and adverse childhood experiences that may have triggered frustration, shame, loss, helplessness, loneliness, or guilt. The impact of such experiences and feelings during formative developmental stages on individuals' perceptions of themselves and others is seen as creating dynamic susceptibilities to depressive disorders, including narcissistic vulnerability, conflicted anger, excessively high expectations of self and others, and maladaptive defense mechanisms. I will briefly review these theories and then use them to distill a core set of psychodynamic factors central to the understanding and treatment of depression. I will then present a case to illustrate the relevance of and approaches to these dynamics.

5.3   Early Psychoanalytic Models of Depression: Disappointment, Loss, and Anger

Early psychoanalytic writers who addressed depression focused on temperamental factors, self-esteem sensitivity, early life adverse events, current losses and disappointments, and conflicted anger (Abraham, 1911, 1924; Freud, 1917) (Rado, 1928). Abraham (1911, 1924) provided an initial analytic framework when he described depression as resulting from hostility toward others that becomes self-directed, a notion that has remained a core dynamic in the view of most psychoanalytic clinicians. He believed depressed patients demonstrated a propensity, based on temperament or early adverse experiences, toward hatred and mistrust of others (Abraham, 1911). Frightened and guilty about their anger, such patients repress their hostility and project it externally. They then feel hated by others and explain this dislike as being caused by their deficiencies or negative attributes.

Based on his observations comparing bereavement and the depressed state (melancholia), Freud (1917) subsequently hypothesized that an important loss in the individual's life, either in reality or in fantasy, can trigger the onset of depression. As distinct from mourning, depression is triggered when the patient has intensely ambivalent feelings about the person (or object, or concept) who is lost. The depressed individual identifies with, or takes on as part of himself or herself, one or some of the lost person's characteristics, to maintain a feeling of connection and to ease feelings of loss. However, because the lost person was viewed with ambivalence, the anger originally directed toward that individual now becomes directed toward the new attributes the patient has adopted. As a result, the patient begins to experience intense self-criticism and self-reproach, which eventually lead to depression.

In a subsequent paper, Abraham (1924), like Freud, posited that anger toward and an identification with the rejecting person leads to a pathological attack on the self. However, he also proposed that current losses or disappointments that trigger depression are experienced, usually unconsciously, as a repetition of an early childhood traumatic experience. Childhood adverse events, such as losing a view of the self as a parent's favorite or frustrations in attempting to gain an alliance with the mother against the father (or vice versa), can cause a severe injury to the child's self-esteem. Onset of the illness in adulthood is triggered by a new disappointment, unleashing strong hostile feelings toward those individuals whom the patient views as rejecting.

Rado (1928) further developed the understanding of the dynamics of narcissistic vulnerability and anger in depressed patients. The low self-esteem in patients susceptible to depression leads to an intense craving for attention from others to feel valued and an inability to tolerate disappointment of these needs. Perceived slights and failures of response cause anger and a drop of self-esteem. Rado further posited that these patients have a split perception of self or others as either all good or all bad. In the process of development of depression, the good qualities of the loved one are internalized in the patient's sense of whom he or she would like to be (or the ego ideal), whereas the bad qualities, as in Freud's formulation, become incorporated into the perception of the ego (or self). Anger at the disappointing other is directed toward the self by the superego (the conscience), which punishes the patient for failures to live up to the ego ideal.

5.4   Later Models for Depression: Problems with Self-Esteem Regulation and Aggression

Bibring (1953) amplified Rado's focus on self-esteem regulation and viewed it as more primary to depression than dynamics involving identification and aggression. Low self-esteem, in his model, derives from a gap between the patient's self-view and what he or she would wish to be, or the ego ideal. In Bibring's conception, this sense of failure and low self-esteem stems from early experiences of helplessness involving persistent frustration of a child's dependent needs. Rather than anger toward others and subsequent guilt fueling depression, helplessness triggers self-directed anger. The predisposition toward depression is determined by a constitutional intolerance of frustration, by the severity and extent of situations of helplessness, and by later developmental factors that might confirm the patient's sense of self-disappointment and failure. His and subsequent theories more clearly identify the impact of specific problems in early parenting on self-esteem and anger management, rather than the more universal childhood traumata (e.g., sibling and Oedipal rivalry) described by the early psychoanalysts.

Jacobson (1954, 1971, 1975) proposed that the predisposition to depression derived from a lack of parental acceptance and emotional understanding. These experiences diminish the child's self-esteem, which intensifies ambivalence and aggressive feelings toward the parents, and guilt. Aggression is turned against the self out of guilt and as a defensive strategy to protect the loved person, preventing enactment of hostile impulses. Jacobson believed that to further counteract the negative impact of parental attitudes, the depressed patient develops an excessively perfectionistic ego ideal and a strict superego. The patient blames himself or herself for any attitudes or behaviors that resemble those despised and feared in the parents, a concept similar to Freud's identification theory of self-attack.

Additionally, significant attachment figures are defensively idealized to protect them from aggression and to support the patient's fragile self-esteem. This idealization leads the depressed individual to expect others to do more than they realistically can, leading to recurrent disappointments. Thus, the dependency on an overvalued other and the presence of excessively high self-expectations lead to an unstable and diminished self-esteem and narcissistic vulnerability.

Brenner (1979) focused on conflicts about competitive, sexual, and aggressive wishes as triggers for depression. Patients feel disempowered or castrated as a punishment for these wishes, often out of awareness. Thus, actual or fantasized successes could be a trigger of depression via the need for punishment. Depression itself can function as a punishment or as a means of diminishing a more effective, competitive stance. Anger at the person who is seen as the punishing agent becomes defensively self-directed as the patient adopts a propitiatory stance.

Kohut emphasized the notion that depressive affects, along with feelings of emptiness, in narcissistically vulnerable individuals are derived from traumatically unempathic parenting. These negative feelings intensify when children's emotional experiences are not sensitively mirrored by their primary caretakers, leaving them feeling alone and emotionally empty, and they look for others to idealize and identify with. Somewhat akin to Jacobson's perspective, they develop a compensatory grandiose sense of self that persists into adulthood, while feelings of inadequacy, emptiness, or badness persist. However, recurrent disappointments trigger and exacerbate the underlying low self-esteem. Technical attention to mirroring these patients' feelings and to issues of idealization and devaluation in the transference relationship with the therapist are emphasized (Kohut, 1971).

5.5 Attachment Theory

Attachment theory, as developed by Bowlby (1969, 1980), draws heavily on an ethological and adaptational perspective. Bowlby viewed attachment as a behavioral system essential for survival, and disruptions of attachment, such as loss of a parent, as crucial in the etiology of anxious and depressive disorders. Loss triggers a series of responses, including angry protest, anxiety, mourning, and ultimately, detachment. Disrupted attachments due to insecure and unstable relationships with parents, or to their rejecting and critical behavior, lead to the development of internal models of the self as unlovable and inadequate and of others as unresponsive and punitive. The individual becomes vulnerable to depression in the setting of later experiences of loss or adversity, seeing such losses as signs of failure and expecting little support from others.

Other psychoanalysts have subsequently explored the impact of insecure and disrupted attachment on cognition and emotion. Fonagy and colleagues (1997), for example, have focused on the adverse impact of insecure attachment on the development of *mentalization*, the ability to conceive behavior and motives in the self and others in terms of mental states. A disruption or distortion in this capacity, in the context of insecure attachment, can lead to problems with emotional regulation and expectations of loss, failure, and rejection, which can adversely affect relationships. Preliminary studies suggest that depressed patients suffer from a deficit in mentalization (Fischer-Kern et al., 2008). The capacity to better recognize the motives and emotional states of self and others can aid patients in understanding negative reactions of others and experience them less personally.

5.6 Defense Mechanisms in Depression

Psychoanalytic theorists have considered the possibility that certain defenses (i.e., internal or behavioral means of averting painful feelings or threatening unconscious fantasies) either may be specifically mobilized by depressive feelings or may predispose individuals to the development of depressive syndromes (Brenner, 1979; Jacobson, 1971). The defenses in depressed patients are initially triggered to contend with painfully low self-esteem or intolerably angry fantasies but actually lead to an exacerbation of depression. Thus, anger projected outward, according to Abraham (1911), becomes directed toward the self, whereas efforts to idealize the self or others to cope with low self-esteem eventually lead to further disappointment and devaluation (Jacobson, 1971). Other defenses mentioned specifically by psychoanalytic authors as mobilized to cope with intolerable anger and sadness include denial, passive aggression, reaction formation, and identification with the aggressor.

In a more systematic study by Bloch, Shear, Markowitz, Leon, & Perry (1993), the defense mechanisms used by patients with dysthymic disorder were compared with those of patients with panic disorder, by using the Defense Mechanism Rating Scale (DMRS) (Perry, 1990). The scale, which contains criteria for operationalized assessment for the presence or absence of each defense, is scored by the use of a psychodynamic interview. Two defenses, denial and repression, were found to be used frequently by both patients with panic disorder and patients with dysthymia. Compared with panic disorder patients, those with dysthymia were found to employ higher levels of devaluation, passive aggression, projection, hypochondriasis, acting out, and projective identification.

In the formulation derived from these data by Bloch et al. (1993), depression can occur through directing anger toward the self, expressing anger passively (passive aggression), distorting perceptions of self and others (devaluation, projection), inviting retaliation from others (acting out, passive aggression), or asking for and then rejecting help. Although there has been variability in results (Porcerelli et al., 2009), subsequent studies have generally substantiated the increased presence of these defenses in depressive disorders (Høglend & Perry, 1998).

In individual patients, the clinician should be alert to the characteristic defenses that they employ, particularly to those noted above. Recognizing these defenses helps alter patients' characteristic perceptions of and responses toward others and find more effective ways of coping with their feelings. Identifying defenses also helps to gain access to underlying intrapsychic conflicts that are triggering them (e.g., conflicted anger).

5.7 Parental Perceptions of Depressed Patients

To test the suggestions of many theorists that problematic parental behavior may contribute to the development of depression, some researchers have systematically studied patients' perceptions of parents. These studies (MacKinnon, Henderson, & Andrews, 1993; Parker, 1983; Perris et al., 1986) have generally found that depressed patients, comparted to controls, described less emotional warmth and greater neglect from their parents. MacKinnon et al. (1993) concluded that "rearing practices which deprived the child of love might be an important risk factor predisposing to depression" (p. 174). Although depressed mood could cause a retrospective distortion of memories of parents, studies suggest that improvement in depression does not affect these perceptions (Gerlsma, Das, & Emmelkamp, 1993; Nitta et al., 2008).

These studies are consistent with the notions suggested by several psychoanalytic theorists that early traumatic or adverse events with parents predispose to the development of depression. Alternatively, patients may perceive their parents as being uncaring or rejecting because of a predisposition to feeling rejected. In either case, it is crucial that such internal parental representations be explored to gain an understanding of the patient's depression.

5.8 Central Dynamics of Depression

5.8.1 A Summary

Based on our literature review, and our own clinical work and psychological research on depression, we identified several core dynamics of depression (Table 5.1). A central feature is narcissistic vulnerability, which could also be called self-esteem sensitivity. This vulnerability can derive from several sources, including traumatic or adverse childhood experiences, current stressors, and intrapsychic conflicts (e.g., punishment for competitive wishes). These patients have preexisting feelings of inadequacy or badness and are highly reactive to intrapsychic and environmental triggers. A sense of narcissistic injury predisposes patients toward the experiences of shame, rejection, and anger, which are often important aspects of depressive episodes.

Conflicted anger also plays a key role in the dynamics of depression. This anger can be triggered by narcissistic injury, loss, immense frustration, or a sense of helplessness. Aggression triggers conscious or unconscious guilt, which contributes to self-denigration and self-defeating behaviors that reinforce the depressive cycle.

Thus, aggression is ultimately directed toward the self, in part through guilt. Other sources include hatred projected outward and then experienced as directed toward the self, and aggressive feelings and fantasies directed toward aspects of the self, identified with an ambivalently experienced other. A severe superego can attack

Table 5.1 Central dynamics of depression

Narcissistic vulnerability	
Cause	Early experience or perceptions of loss, rejection, inadequacy, possible biochemical vulnerability
Content	Sensitivity to perceived or actual losses, rejections
Consequences	Recurrent lowering of self-esteem, triggering depressive affects; rage in response to experience of injury
Conflicted anger	
Cause	Response to narcissistic injury; anger at perceived or actual lack of responsiveness of others to the individual's needs and wishes; anger may also arise from blaming of others for one's sense of vulnerability, or being deeply envious of those who seem less vulnerable
Content	Anger at others for injurious, unresponsive behavior, attitudes; blaming others for one's vulnerability; envy of others who are viewed as less vulnerable; anger at others experienced as damaging, threatening, unacceptable, requiring suppression or redirection
Consequences	Disruptions in interpersonal relationships; anger turned toward the self, triggering depressive affects, lowering of self-esteem
Severe superego, experience of guilt and shame	
Cause	Anger turned toward the self via harsh self-judgments; internalization of parental attitudes perceived as harsh and punitive
Content	Anger, greed, envy, sexuality, and accompanying wishes seen as wrong or bad
Consequences	Negative self-perceptions and self-criticisms trigger lowering of self-esteem, depressive affects
Idealized and devalued expectations of self, others	
Cause	Efforts to mitigate low self-esteem
Content	High self-expectations (ego ideal), others idealized in meeting individual's needs, others devalued to bolster self-esteem
Consequences	Significant disappointment, anger at self and others, with lowering of self-esteem
Characteristic means of defending against painful affects (defenses)	
Cause	Intolerable feelings of low self-esteem, anger
Content	Denial, projection (seeing anger as coming from others), passive aggression (expressing anger indirectly), reaction formation (denial of anger accompanied by compensatory overly positive feelings)
Consequences	Anger not effectively dealt with; increased depression via anger directed toward the self or via the world seen as hostile, menacing, uncaring, or defeating

the self for various aggressive, competitive, and sexual feelings, lowering self-esteem.

Depressed patients often attempt to modulate self-esteem and aggression via idealization and devaluation, leading to increased susceptibility to depression when the responses of idealized others prove to be disappointing. An overly perfectionistic ego ideal and superego develops in an attempt to compensate for low self-esteem. Patients fail to live up to these narcissistic aspirations and moral expectations, leading to a loss of self-esteem.

Finally, characteristic defenses, such as denial, projection, passive aggression, and reaction formation, represent a means of warding off painful depressive affects but often result in an increase in depression.

5.9   A Core Dynamic Formulation for Depression

Psychodynamic literature, studies, and clinical work, then, suggest two broad models of depression: those involving aggression toward others that is ultimately directed toward the self and those focusing on difficulties with self-esteem in patients whose expectations of themselves and others far exceed the capacity to live up to them. Finally, the two models can be linked. These two core dynamic aspects for depression typically trigger vicious cycles. In each formulation, narcissistic vulnerability and low self-esteem are seen as fundamental to the susceptibility to depression.

In depression cycle 1 (Fig. 5.1), this vulnerability results in sensitivity to disappointment and rejection and thus to easily triggered rage. The anger causes conflict and/or is experienced as damaging, causing feelings of guilt and badness. The self-directed rage compounds the injury to self-esteem, which then escalates the narcissistic vulnerability, and so on, in a vicious cycle. Defenses, including denial, projection, passive aggression, identification with the aggressor, and reaction formation, are triggered in an attempt to diminish these painful feelings but result in an intensification of depression. Precipitants for depression can include perceived or actual loss or rejection, the failure to live up to a perfectionistic ego ideal, and superego punishment for sexual and aggressive fantasies.

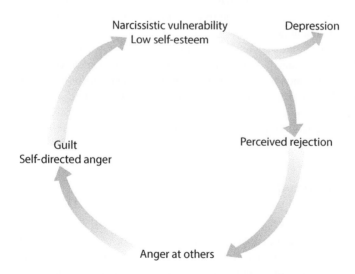

Fig. 5.1 Vicious cycle 1 in depression: narcissistic vulnerability and anger

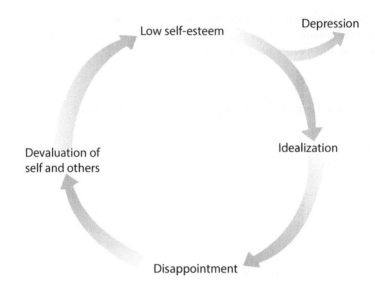

Fig. 5.2 Vicious cycle 2 in depression: low self-esteem and idealization/devaluation

Another core dynamic in depression (depression cycle 2) is the individual's attempt to deal with low self-esteem by idealization and devaluation (Fig. 5.2). Feelings of inadequacy or helplessness will lead to compensatory idealization of self or others, increasing the likelihood and intensity of eventual disappointment, triggering depression. An ego ideal with highly unrealistic standards develops, increasing the level of disappointment with and devaluation of the self when these standards cannot be met. Alternately, individuals may devalue others to maintain self-esteem, but the aggression in this stance triggers superego punishment. In addition, aggressive behavior may lead to the patient's alienating others, adding to feelings of abandonment and rejection.

As noted above, the two sets of dynamics also interact with each other, because conflicts over self-esteem and anger can heighten the tendency toward idealization and devaluation, and disappointments following idealization can lead to anger, guilt, and self-criticism. Although these cycles represent core dynamics of depression, clinicians should not restrict themselves to these factors and should remain alert to other areas of vulnerability, intrapsychic conflict, and defense.

5.10   Case Example

Mr. A was a 46-year-old White businessman who presented with about 4 months of down mood and disruptions in mood, energy, sleep, and concentration, with no suicidal ideation. The therapist recommended an antidepressant trial, but the patient was fearful of side effects and wanted to see whether therapy alone might work.

They agreed to proceed with psychodynamic psychotherapy, keeping medication in mind as an option. In exploring the context of symptom onset, Mr. A described how his depression was triggered after one of his stores abruptly closed. The closure was necessary after an important backer, a former mentor, withdrew support, which deeply upset the patient:

Mr. A: I don't get why John did this. I've really admired his business skills, best in the profession. He's been helpful with advice when I was anxious about some deals. So it's really disturbing that he would pull his support so suddenly. I don't get it, and I've felt devastated.

Th: It sounds terrible that somebody whom you admired so much pulled out like this. Did he explain to you why he changed his mind?

Mr. A: No. Just the generic "needing to go in another direction."

Th: Are you mad at him?

Mr. A: Maybe a little bit but mostly at myself. What did I do to screw this up? What did I do that caused him to withdraw? It makes no sense.

During this evaluation phase, the outlines of the dynamics of Mr. A's depression were already emerging. He was deeply injured by the withdrawal of a man he idealized for his business skills and emotional support. However, instead of being angry at John, he blamed himself, believing he must have done something "bad" that caused John's action. He became catastrophic, frightened that "my whole business is going to fall apart," even though he owned several stores and was losing just one of them. Indeed, he was already in touch with another potential backer. Rather than feeling relieved by this reality, Mr. A was already caught in the cycles of depression. He was deeply hurt and his self-esteem injured by the withdrawal of his friend and believed he did not live up to his own business standards; his anger at John became directed toward himself. The therapist worked to clarify the sources of his bleak view of himself and the future:

Th: I think we need to examine the intensity of your self-criticism and your fears, because you view yourself as much more of a failure and worried about the future than the circumstances call for. Overall your business continues to do very well! Let's talk about your history to see if that might help us to understand your reactions better.

Mr. A described his childhood as positive only until the birth of his sister at age 5. He remembered feeling angry and jealous about the attention that she received. At some point, he somehow became viewed as the "bad" child and his sister was "the good one." He felt isolated and lonely in response to his parents' attacks, as they sometimes would not speak to him for a day or two in response to his behavior. In reviewing what he actually did, it emerged that many of the criticisms were about his tendency toward assertiveness and taking chances that actually subsequently aided him in his business ventures. For instance, at age 14, he took his father's car for a spin without telling them. He was grounded for 2 weeks but also was castigated for being a "rotten" kid who "would come to no good." As an adolescent, he pushed curfews and often avoided his studies, leading to his parents' opprobrium, in part to work in stores where he gained valuable experience. None of his actual behavior explained the degree to which he felt his parents perceived him as "bad" and favored his sister. As therapy progressed, the patient realized that his parents were highly rigid, conservative people heavily influenced by their own traumatic histories, including growing up in poverty. They were extremely careful about money, which he spent more freely. They criticized him for not getting a "regular" job, by which they meant a doctor or lawyer. Indeed, the patient's freedom with expenditures and his entrepreneurial attitude helped to gain ownership of his first store at age 25.

As Mr. A proceeded with his career, he greatly admired what he considered to be "titans" of real estate, of whom John was one. He worked for them in lower level positions in an effort to learn their approaches and be more connected to them. He idealized them, and even after his own successes, devalued himself by comparison, viewing himself as a minor player. "I'm not really in the big leagues. I've had some accomplishments, but they really pale in comparison to these guys." The therapist continued to address Mr. A's devaluation and self-blame, in part by encouraging mentalization:

Mr. A: I still don't get why John pulled out. I keep obsessing about it. I assume he thinks I've made some bad decisions. But I don't know what those could be.
Th: What makes you think he pulled out based on what you did rather than some other reason of his own?
Mr. A: It feels that way. But I know how he works, and he doesn't tend to let personal matters cloud his decisions. He probably needed the money for a bigger venture. But I'm worried when this gets around people are going to think there's something bad about me or my business.
Th: That designation sounds very familiar from your childhood.
Mr. A: Yes that's true.
Th: I believe part of why his withdrawal hurts so much is because you really idealized him to make up for bad feelings you had about yourself, and because you felt he really understood you. He recognized your business acumen. That makes it all the more disappointing now that he's pulled back.
Mr. A: I did overestimate him. I mean I never would have expected he would behave in this way.

Mr. A's dynamics identified in this phase of treatment are consistent with depression cycle 2, in which his self-esteem vulnerability led to idealized expectations of himself and others, creating a precipitous drop in mood when he was disillusioned and felt like a failure. Although actually a minor disruption of his business, symbolically his mentor's withdrawal and closure of the store represented a significant loss of an idealized other. The patient often experienced these emotional threats in financial terms, fueling irrational catastrophic concerns about his business.

Although he was deeply disappointed by John's withdrawal, Mr. A initially denied being angry at him: "I'm sure he had a reason for doing this." He focused more on blaming himself. However, as the idealization was addressed, he began to more realistically assess his friend, and became more aware of his anger:

Mr. A: I guess one thing I don't understand is why he didn't tell me about this move before making it. What would have been the problem with that? And that at least would give me some time to prepare for what happened. I wouldn't have been caught up short.

Th: Well I know you previously denied being frustrated but as you talk you really sound quite mad at him. Particularly about the way he handled it.

Mr. A: I do see what you're saying. And maybe I am becoming more aware of being angry. I was just blaming myself for what happened.

Th: According to the idea of you being the bad one.

Mr. A: Yeah, but the more I think about it, the more I feel he could have worked with me. I mean he could have told me what he thought the problem was, and I could have addressed it. Or he could have said "there's no problem: I just need to use the money for a new venture." And he did create a lot of trouble for me, unnecessarily.

Th: I think you have been suppressing a lot of your anger and directing it at yourself.

Mr. A: I think that's true but that's changing.

In this vignette, Mr. A demonstrated the dynamics of depression cycle 1. His anger at others was a source of conflict and he was frightened about the damage it would cause. He ended up unconsciously directing this anger at himself in the form of guilt, self-criticism, and a sense of badness. The trigger for his depression involved the loss of his relationship with an idealized figure, an old mentor. As described by Abraham, this loss also triggered dynamics related to painful feelings from his childhood, including the birth of his sister and his role as the "bad one" in the family. Mr. A had rageful reactions in response to these disappointments, but they were expressed unconsciously and directed toward himself.

It also emerged that Mr. A felt guilty about his competitive wishes (see Brenner above), and he experienced John's withdrawal as punishment. This guilt was linked to the intensity of the anger he felt toward his sister for being the focus of his parents' attention. Easing the threat from his competitive wishes diminished his guilt about assertiveness, helping to increase his efforts on his own behalf. This shift also enabled him to be more comfortable recognizing his own success, further reducing his narcissistic vulnerability.

In treatment of Mr. A, the therapist identified how he idealized his old mentor and other real estate "titans," and this connection helped to bolster his low self-esteem. These idealizing fantasies set him up for disappointment with others and an overly negative view of his own competence, believing he was not capable of achieving their level of success. The therapist highlighted these excessive self-expectations, helping him to develop a more realistic sense of his success relative to others. This shift in perceptions also helped to relieve his view of himself as "bad."

Additionally, identifying his anger at others led to conscious recognition and greater tolerance of these feelings. He came to believe that anger at his parents and his old mentor were justified and felt less threatened by it. This eased his propensity to direct anger at himself, including viewing himself as "bad." He recognized that he was reprimanding himself as his parents did, despite disagreeing with their perception of him. In addition, better management of his anger reduced the need to idealize others as a way of protecting them from his feelings.

References

Abraham, K. (1911/1927). Notes on the psycho-analytical investigation and treatment of manic depressive insanity and allied conditions. In *Selected papers on psychoanalysis* (pp. 137–156). London: Hogarth Press.

Abraham, K. (1924/1927). A short study of the development of the libido, viewed in the light of mental disorders. In *Selected papers on psychoanalysis* (pp. 418–501). London: Hogarth Press.

American Psychiatric Association. (2010). Practice guideline for the treatment of patients with major depressive disorder (Third edition). *The American Journal of Psychiatry, 157*(Suppl), 1–45.

Bibring, E. (1953). The mechanics of depression. In P. Greenacre (Ed.), *Affective disorders: Psychoanalytic contributions to their study* (pp. 13–48). New York, NY: International Universities Press.

Bloch, A. L., Shear, M. K., Markowitz, J. C., Leon, A. C., & Perry, J. C. (1993). An empirical study of defense mechanisms in dysthymia. *The American Journal of Psychiatry, 150*(8), 1194–1198.

Bowlby, J. (1969). *Attachment and loss, Vol 1: Attachment*. New York, NY: Basic Books.

Bowlby, J. (1980). *Attachment and loss, Vol 3: Loss*. New York, NY: Basic Books.

Brenner, C. (1979). Depressive affect, anxiety, and psychic conflict in the phallic-oedipal phase. *The Psychoanalytic Quarterly, 48*(2), 177–197.

Busch, F. N. (2018). *Psychodynamic approaches to behavioral change*. Arlington, VA: American Psychiatric Press.

Busch, F. N., Milrod, B. L., Chen, C. K., & Singer, M. (in press). *Trauma-focused psychodynamic psychotherapy*. Oxford: Oxford University Press.

Busch, F. N., Milrod, B. L., Singer, M., & Aronson, A. (2012). *Panic-focused psychodynamic psychotherapy, extended range*. New York, NY: Routledge.

Busch, F. N., Rudden, M. G., & Shapiro, T. (2016). *Psychodynamic treatment of depression* (2nd ed.). Arlington, VA: American Psychiatric Press.

CANMAT. (2016). 2016 Clinical guidelines for the management of adults with major depressive disorder. *The Canadian Journal of Psychiatry, 61*(9), 504–603.

Driessen, E., Cuijpers, P., de Maat, S. C., Abbass, A. A., de Jonghe, F., & JJM, D. (2010). The efficacy of short-term psychodynamic psychotherapy for depression: A meta-analysis. *Clinical Psychology Review, 30*(1), 25–36.

Eaton, W. W., Shao, H., Nestadt, G., Lee, H. B., Bienvenu, O. J., & Zandi, P. (2008). Population-based study of first onset and chronicity in major depressive disorder. *Archives of General Psychiatry, 65*(5), 513–520.

Fischer-Kern, M., Tmej, A., Kapusta, N. D., Naderer, A., Leithner-Dziubas, K., Löffler-Stastka, H., & Springer-Kremser, M. (2008). The capacity for mentalization in depressive patients: A pilot study. *Zeitschrift für Psychosomatische Medizin und Psychotherapie, 54*, 368–380.

Fonagy, P., & Target, M. (1997). Attachment and reflective function: Their role in self-organization. *Development and Psychopathology, 9*(4), 679–700.

Freud, S. (1917/1957). Mourning and melancholia. In J. Strachey (Ed. & Trans.), *The standard edition of the complete psychological works of Sigmund Freud* (Vol. 14, pp. 239–258). London: Hogarth Press.

Gerlsma, C., Das, J., & Emmelkamp, P. M. (1993). Depressed patients' parental representations: Stability across changes in depressed mood and specificity across diagnoses. *Journal of Affective Disorders, 27*(3), 173–181.

Høglend, P., & Perry, J. C. (1998). Defensive functioning predicts improvement in major depressive episodes. *The Journal of Nervous and Mental Disease, 186*(4), 238–243.

Jacobson, E. (1954). Transference problems in the psychoanalytic treatment of severely depressed patients. *Journal of the American Psychoanalytic Association, 2*, 695–705.

Jacobson, E. (1971). *Depression: Comparative studies of normal, neurotic, and psychotic conditions.* New York, NY: International Universities Press.

Jacobson, E. (1975). The psychoanalytic treatment of depressive patients. In B. Anthony (Ed.), *Depression and human existence* (pp. 431–443). Boston, MA: Little, Brown.

Judd, L. L., Akiskal, H. S., & Paulus, M. P. (1997). The role and clinical significance of subsyndromal depressive symptoms (SSD) in unipolar major depressive disorder. *Journal of Affective Disorders, 45*(1–2), 5–17., discussion 17–18.

Keller, M. B., Hanks, D. L., & Klein, D. N. (1996). Summary of the DSM-IV mood disorders field trial and issue overview. *The Psychiatric Clinics of North America, 19*(1), 1–28.

Kocsis, J. H., & Klein, D. N. (Eds.). (1995). *Diagnosis and treatment of chronic depression.* New York, NY: Guilford.

Kohut, H. (1971). *The analysis of the self.* New York, NY: International Universities Press.

Leichsenring, F., Leweke, F., Klein, S., & Steinert, C. (2015). The empirical status of psychodynamic psychotherapy—An update: Bambi's alive and kicking. *Psychotherapy and Psychosomatics, 84*(3), 129–148.

MacKinnon, A., Henderson, A. S., & Andrews, G. (1993). Parental 'affectionless control' as an antecedent to adult depression: A risk factor refined. *Psychological Medicine, 23*(1), 135–141.

Nitta, M., Narita, T., Umeda, K., Hattori, M., Naitoh, H., & Iwata, N. (2008). Influence of negative cognition on the parental bonding instrument (PBI) in patients with major depression. *The Journal of Nervous and Mental Disease, 196*(3), 244–246.

Parker, G. (1983). Parental 'affectionless control' as an antecedent to adult depression. A risk factor delineated. *Archives of General Psychiatry, 40*(9), 956–960.

Perris, C., Arrindell, W. A., Perris, H., Eisemann, M., van der Ende, J., & von Knorring, J. (1986). Perceived depriving parental rearing and depression. *The British Journal of Psychiatry, 148*, 170–175.

Perry, J. C. (1990). *The defense mechanism rating scales* (5th ed.). Cambridge, MA: Author.

Porcerelli, J. H., Olson, T. R., Presniak, M. D., Markava, T., & Miller, K. (2009). Defense mechanisms and major depressive disorder in African American women. *The Journal of Nervous and Mental Disease, 197*(10), 736–714.

Rado, S. (1928). The problem of melancholia. *The International Journal of Psycho-Analysis, 9*, 420–438.

Vieta, E., Sánchez-Moreno, J., Lahuerta, J., Zaragoza, S., & EDHIPO Group (Hypomania Detection Study Group). (2008). Subsyndromal depressive symptoms in patients with bipolar and unipolar disorder during clinical remission. *Journal of Affective Disorders, 107*(1–3), 169–174.

Chapter 6
Case Study of a 44-Year-Old Patient with a Moderate Recurrent Depressive Disorder (ICD-10 F 33.1) from Psychodynamic Point of View

Christos Charis

Contents

6.1 Introduction

Mrs. X is a 44-year-old divorced mother of one (daughter) who presented with a major depression of moderate intensity which was already chronic as she came to me for therapy (09/17). The onset of the depression was present when Mrs. X was 34 years old. She decided to rent a flat with her boyfriend who she loved. She developed severe panic attacks at that moment and became very depressed. Again, Mrs. X became severely depressed at the age of 41. The patient had a course of electroconvulsive therapy (ECT, 22 electroshocks) and after that behaviour therapy for 1 year. All those treatments helped her to feel better, but she felt exhausted every day and had a low mood. The psychodynamic analysis showed two conflicts, a narcissistic conflict and an autonomous-dependent conflict, as they are defined in the Operationalized Psychodynamic Diagnosis-2 (OPD-2) (Arbeitskreis, 2006). These conflicts are due to the treatment of Mrs. X by her parents and because of her disappointing experiences when she had to escape from her own country when she was 13 years old. She had to act against her own will. We can analyse the psychodynamics of Mrs. X with regard to the concept of Sidney Blatt, a psychoanalyst (Blatt & Blass, 1996; Blatt, Luyten, & Corveleyn, 2005). Blatt investigated areas that

C. Charis (✉)
Private Practice, Dillenburg, Germany

© Springer Nature Switzerland AG 2021
C. Charis, G. Panayiotou (eds.), *Depression Conceptualization and Treatment*,
https://doi.org/10.1007/978-3-030-68932-2_6

concern the everyday experiences of depressive people. The first core theme is "loneliness, weakness, helplessness and abandonment. Desires to be cared for, loved and protected". This factor was called "dependency" or "anaclitic". The second factor is preoccupation with self-definitional areas ("introjective": harsh self-criticism; perfectionism). Introjective depression is characterized by a tendency towards self-criticism and self-evaluation. Our patient did not learn to trust other people because of her very disappointing experiences with her parents. This led to a very weak self-consciousness and an excessively perfectionistic ego ideal. These traits have played an important role for the onset of chronic depression of Mrs. X. The depressive symptoms of Mrs. X have been relieved even more in a psychodynamic treatment which is ongoing. (Until July 2020, 90 sessions have taken place.) She has succeeded in partially reducing her demands on herself.

6.2   Theoretical Digression

We can analyse the psychodynamics of Mrs. X with regard to the concept of Sidney Blatt, a psychoanalyst and a professor at Yale University in the USA (Blatt et al., 2005; Blatt & Blass, 1996). Taking this concept into account, he sifted through the classical psychoanalytical literature (Bibring, 1952; Cohen et al., 1954; Freud, 1916–1917), and from the study of this literature, he investigated areas that concern the everyday experiences of depressive people and their families instead of depressive symptoms. On this basis, he was able to formulate 66 items ("Depressive Experiences Questionnaire") and present them to a large sample of students. The main component analysis with varimax rotation revealed two primary factors (Blatt, D'Afflitti, & Quinlan, 1976). The first core theme is "loneliness, weakness, helplessness and abandonment. Desires to be cared for, loved and protected". People like this worry about the danger of losing somebody (most especially important persons) from among their group. They primarily deal with problems in interpersonal relatedness. This factor was called "dependency" or "anaclitic" (fears of abandonment; dependency). The second factor is preoccupied with self-definitional areas ("introjective": harsh self-criticism; perfectionism). Introjective depression is characterized by a tendency towards self-criticism and self-evaluation. These people are busy with their lives and have feelings of guilt because they find themselves unable to live up to standards. They say, for example, "There is a big difference between the way I am at the moment and the way I would like to be". This coincides with Freud's view of "the sources" of a depression, namely, superego conflicts against the background of an unstable self-esteem and problems in the interpersonal realm with feelings of loneliness and fears of abandonment (Blatt, 1998, 2004, 2005). These findings agree both with psychoanalytical theories (e.g. Arieti & Bemporad, 1980) and with behavioural theories (Beck, 1983). Many studies from different cultures have shown that these research results are extremely stable (e.g. Beutel et al., 2004; Luyten, 2002). There is an ongoing debate on the relevance of this theoretical model (e.g. Blatt et al., 2005; Reis & Grenyer, 2002). In support of it, perfectionism as a distinguishing quality was repeatedly found to be associated with a more problematic course in depression. Overall, it can be assumed that personality characteristics and other patient traits (social support, interpersonal problems, etc.) not only are overall predictors of outcome but also interact with the form of treatment or setting provided. In any case, it is important to distinguish between depressions focused on interpersonal and self-value issues (Blatt & Maroudas, 1992). The close relationships that addict-depressives maintain are related to their fears of rejection, so that they behave demandingly and staunchly, annoying others, so that they end up being rejected: what they originally feared. Relationships of perfectionist subtypes are characterized by rivalry and ambivalence, so that they awaken criticisms in significant others! Factor analysis studies indicate that there is an adaptive or "healthy" perfectionism and a misadapted or "unhealthy" perfectionism (Enns, Cox, & Clara, 2002). Obviously, anaclitic subtype and perfectionist-depressed people develop mental representations of themselves and others against this background, which regularly lead to the dreaded interactions in the same way. Therefore, the therapy should focus on these mental representations of the self and the important others (Blatt et al., 2005; Shahar & Mayes, 2017).

6.3   Biography

The 44-year-old divorced patient (Mrs. X) has been living with her boyfriend (47) and her 25-year-old daughter in a city in Germany in her newly purchased apartment for half a year. She and her daughter moved from another town 2 years ago to his rented apartment.

She grew up in another country until she turned 13, after which she reluctantly emigrated to Germany with her parents. Her parents had not prepared her or informed her about their plan to emigrate, which still has an impact on her life today. She has the feeling of being betrayed by her parents.

Mrs. X experienced her mother who gave birth to her at the age of 23 while studying chemistry as someone who still wants to take over decisions about her daughter and give her advice; thus, she rebelled against her. Her father (+34, store man) was bad-tempered, but very reliable. He spent some time with her doing activities for children. Both parents had to work; hence, her grandmother had to look after her during their absence. Mrs. X was very affectionate to her.

In addition, memories from her childhood are missing. During her first year in Germany, Mrs. X had great language difficulties in the school because she did not speak German before; nevertheless, she made great progress at the end of the school year. She moved to high school but she did not achieve the high school certificate. She had little confidence in herself to pass it. Her dream job was to become a physiotherapist which she trained for; it took her 3 years. She worked as a physiotherapist for 6 years in a big hospital; she was dissatisfied, because they required hard work. In her work, she got to meet a colleague. He was the first relationship after her failed marriage. He wanted to marry her and have children with her. She loved him;

he looked the way she really liked. When she went on holiday with him and her daughter for the first time, she experienced dizziness in the dining room of the hotel, could not feel her legs anymore and could not walk safely. The holiday meant for her making a decision to start a new life, she told me. And when she signed the contract for the shared flat, Mrs. X had her first panic attack. She also became depressed. She broke up the relationship. Since her job gradually begun to burden her, she has retrained to become a "healthcare clerk". She completed her course in 2 years instead of the normal 3 years with a very good A grade and in this time had a job as a cleaning lady. Immediately after completing this retraining, she took up a degree in "Health and Social Care" but without a final exam because shortly before that (2015) she became severely depressed again. The study during her training phase got her to the new position as a healthcare professional, which meant she was studying and working. She went to a university every single weekend for 2 years for her lessons. In the second year, she became very depressed (2015). She was very ill for a long time and unable to work for 7 months. She received 22 ECTs in a psychiatric hospital. She had a treatment in cognitive behavioural therapy for a year without improvement, she told me.

In 1995 (20), she had married a man her age from her country (a locksmith). Her husband was an alcoholic and drug addict. Because she did not receive any child support for their daughter after separation, her parents urged her to get back with him, but they quarrelled very often. In 2003, she left him.

6.4 Psychodynamics

Mrs. X has a very ambivalent relationship with her mother who was her primary caretaker. The mother of Mrs. X has a very dominant personality and she loves to give advice to everybody. The behavior of her mother leads Mrs. X to believe that she cannot please her, because no matter how she does it, she always gets advice from her. But she wants to be seen by her mother the other way around. Mrs. X wants to feel the ordinary loving care of her mother and less her advice. She wishes to hear from her mother, for example, the following words: "Bravo you are doing that very well! (see Table 6.1)".

Because of those experiences, she develops a feeling of helplessness which she experiences every day in her relationships with other people. These experiences and feelings put a pressure on Mrs. X, who believes, because she is not good enough, she must do more. She became in that way a perfectionist and achievement-oriented. She cannot trust so easily and she is afraid of closeness because she felt like she

Table 6.1 Psychodynamic

The patient experienced her mother as:
Very dominant, giving advice all the time, less loving, strong, guilty of betraying (because of the emigration when she was 13)

would be injured and disappointed. We can recognize these fears in her dreams. For example, she is in a high building. Although she is alone and is very scared, she dares to go higher. In another dream, she goes to the USA alone although she cannot speak English. She manages to find work and is beginning to work there. Another example of her perfectionistic tendency is the fact that she learned German very well within 1 year so that she could go to the German high school. Her perfectionism was an important reason for the second episode of depression. Mrs. X began a new job and at the same time she began to study. Besides that, she landed a cleaning work. On the other hand, she admires her mother for her strength. Her mother, for example, studied chemistry and is very ambitious. Because of that, she has begun a process of identification with her mother and she is developing a similar relationship to her daughter. She sees her daughter only as her daughter and not as an autonomous person and that they have a symbiotic relationship. Because Mrs. X does not have a clear idea of what autonomy is, when her daughter tried to detach herself from her mother (her daughter wanted to go abroad after finishing her high school), Mrs. X tried also to detach herself from her own mother. She got to know her current boyfriend and she moved with him in another Bundesland, but she is not autonomous enough to cope with that development. She became dependent again on her boyfriend. Her boyfriend tries to help her. He introduces her to his friends. And he wants to get married to her, but she does not agree with the idea. She only agreed to get married to him when she has got enough money. That means she is afraid to get more dependent on him. She is afraid to become disappointed again because if she gets married to him, an even more close relationship will flourish. And because of that, she does not like sex. Sex means closeness with somebody. She is afraid of closeness because she can be injured and disappointed. Her friend has already injured her as he told her he loves her in a moderate way. Besides that, she has been injured by her mother who began to work when Mrs. X was a baby. Furthermore, her mother and her father brought her to Germany without speaking with her about that; they did not ask Mrs. X whether she wants to stay in her country or to come to Germany, because in the first place, she really did not want to come to Germany. Thus, she lost her grandmother in that way. She has been disappointed until today because of that. Her mother did not show her affection. And because of that, Mrs. X has been very angry with her mother, but she cannot show her anger because she depends on her. That means she needs her mother. Therefore, she tries to do everything alone. She believes the following: "If I accept a close relationship, then I will be injured. I will be disappointed because I cannot trust the important others in my life. They have all disappointed me always!" But because she is not satisfied with that solution, she came for therapy. The position of our patient in her life is as follows: "I keep people who try to come near me away. In that way I can stay autonomous; nobody can injure me. But she is not really autonomous! She depends on her mother". She belongs to the group of the self-defining autonomous according to Blatt's configuration (see Table 6.2).

Therefore, we can understand the conversion symptoms of our patient in that way: She was on vacation with her boyfriend at that time and her decision to take that holiday with him was her conscious decision to intensify the relationship with

Table 6.2 Psychodynamic

• All those experiences with her mother have had a great influence on the mental and social development of the patient
• Because she admires her mother for her strength, she begins a process of identification with her mother and cannot detach from her mother. She develops a similar relationship with her daughter. Due to that dependency on her mother, she is very angry with her, but cannot show it. In relationships with significant others, she is scared of getting dependent on them. Because of that, she has problems with sex. She tries to do everything alone. But she is pseudoautonomous
She grew up having a feeling of not being good enough. She became perfectionist ("mental representations of oneself")

Table 6.3 Psychodynamic

• The patient became ill (panic attacks and depression)
• For the first time in 2008 when she signed the contract for the shared flat. Why? Because she believed that if she gets married to him and she has kids with him, she will become very dependent on him. Since he will disappoint her—according to her experiences with significant others (her parents and later her husband)—she is panic-stricken by this dependency
• The patient told me: "I thought if I get married to him and have children, I will make myself extremely dependent on him! Then I will be completely blocked! I will not be able to act!" She feels completely helpless!

Table 6.4 Psychodynamic

• The patient became severly depressed 2014
• For this second episode of depression
• Her perfectionism was an important reason. Mrs. X began a new work and at the same time she began to study (she went to a university every single weekend for 2 years for lesson). Besides that, she charred. She overtaxed herself with all that

him. Because of that, she took her daughter with them. But she cannot intensify the relationship with him because she is unconsciously afraid that if she lets somebody come near her, she will be injured. She has learned this through her experiences with significant others, e.g., her parents, through her life. She is now afraid that if she takes that step, she will be disappointed by the significant others, in that case her boyfriend. Therefore, she could not walk confidently in the dining room of the hotel where she was with her boyfriend. And because of that, she got panic attacks when she wanted to sign the rental agreement for the flat to live with him. She became very ill! She got panic attacks and she became depressed, because she believed that if she gets married to him and she has kids with him, she will make herself very dependent on him. Since he will disappoint her—according to her experiences with important others—she is panic-stricken by this dependency. Those are her fears against another disappointment from a significant other as she knows that through her experiences with her parents and later her husband. The patient told me: "I thought if I get married to him and have children I will make myself extremely dependent on him! Then I will be completely blocked! I will not be able to act!" She feels completely helpless! (see Tables 6.3 and 6.4).

6.5   Therapy

This therapy began on the initiative of Mrs. X and on the advice of the psychosomatic hospital where she had been treated before this therapy started. Mrs. X came to me in September 2017 on the advice of her boyfriend, who had been in my therapy in the past. I think she chose me as her therapist because she saw that the therapy of her boyfriend was successful. I think it was also important for her that I am a migrant in Germany as she is. I suppose she hoped I would understand her better than somebody else. That means she identified herself with me and in that way she felt stronger in order to feel less damaged or vulnerable. It is possible that she came to me as a psychodynamic therapist because she was disappointed with the behaviour therapy. That is a common phenomenon: Patients who are not satisfied with the direction of one type of therapy change the form of therapy when they need therapy again. I decided to accept her in my therapy for different reasons. First, I suggested to her boyfriend that if she wanted she could become my patient. I did not want to disappoint either of them. In addition, I found her pleasant and intelligent. Those are good conditions for a successful therapy. I had the impression she is suitable for such a therapy. I found it remarkable that she was persuaded from the beginning of the therapy that I was the right therapist for her. It was very difficult to believe that I could help her feel more at ease with herself, to be more in touch with her feelings.

She reported in the first session about her condition: She feels quite exhausted all the time, and she feels numb! She feels turmoil, but she can't let it out. All of this makes her tired and she has nightmares. One her nightmares is as follows: She is not allowed to enter her house in her home country. She could not come to terms with that situation. She explained to me that she came to Germany with her parents when she was 13, in her puberty. Her looking back in consternation was easy to understand. She said she could not understand anything here because she could not speak German and she had to go to school immediately after coming here! And then she told me she learned the German language within a year and so she could move to high school. I understood from the patient's explanation that she was seeking my approval. She reported more about her life, about the history of the relationship with her boyfriend as I have written it in the biography (s. there). She became very ill when she wanted to sign the rental agreement. She got panic attacks and she became severely depressed. She could not sleep anymore. Because of her complaints, she decided to leave her boyfriend, although she still loved him, after 5 years. She is focusing her attention on her parents and her relationship to them. She told me she would like to have a closer relationship with her mother. In an interaction with her mother, we can see her emotional needs, i.e. emotional support including the provision of love and a sense of belonging. Mrs. X would like to buy a specific armchair for her flat. She phones her mother and requests if she could look for such a chair in the big city where she lives. I am pointing out the behaviour of Mrs. X: "Have you noticed that it is important for you to ask your mother for help whereas you could find that on your own?" (We call that confrontation in the psychodynamic therapy.) She did not answer and she smiled at my challenge. She had a dream after that. She had that dream at a time at which she is looking for a flat to buy. In the dream, she bought the flat, but the flat is in the same city where her mother lives. (Mrs. X lives really somewhere completely different from her mother.) I used an interpretation in that phase of treatment. "I see your ambivalence in that dream regarding buying a flat. You want consciously to be with your boyfriend and want to buy an apartment with him, but unconsciously you want to be near your mother". She answered, "Yes, that is right. I am realizing now how difficult it is to let go of my parents". She admitted that if she is planning something, she asks herself what her parents will think about that. When she visited her parents with her boyfriend, her boyfriend mentioned that her mother acts as a guardian for her. Mrs. X answers that her boyfriend is right. She lets her mother interfere a lot in her life. She remembers several situations where she did not do what she wanted but she did what their parents wanted. For example, she stayed as a physiotherapist in a big hospital although she would have liked to leave because she had been working very hard there. When the hospital offered her a severance payment, she did not accept it because her parents did not want that. That was not their own opinion. For the same reason, she got married to her husband because her parents urged her to get married. They are Catholics. It is important for them, when a man and a woman live together, that they are married. She was 20 years old at that time and she did not want to get married. When she divorced him, she went back to her parents and lived with them. Her parents looked after her then. (Then she compared herself with her daughter. She mentioned her daughter is more independent than her; for example, her daughter has decided to go abroad soon. Mrs. X is worried about her daughter, but she knows that she denies her own feelings and instead perceives her fears as coming from her daughter.) And then she said: "Everybody should visit their parents once a month! She aimed to please her parents in that way!" I asked her if something like that was not stressful. (We call that "clarification".) By that formulation, I try to point out the dependence of the patient on her mother without increasing her resistance to the uncovering therapy. She answered that I was right. I asked her if she wanted to please her parents for entirely altruistic motives or if she derived some benefits herself. She smiled and told me it was important for her to have somebody who was interested in her and loved her. But she is trying to free herself from the bonds with her parents in order to liberate herself from her relationship with her boyfriend. She explained to me that although she believed she would quarrel with him, she agreed to buy a house with him. That means her wish for attachment and family is stronger than her fears of being hurt by significant others if she allows them to get closer to her. As a therapist, I asked myself how we can explain this progressive development of the patient. Possibly, she is affected by her experiences in the therapy. Perhaps her experiences with me are like a bridge for her to let somebody else get closer to her, because she experienced me as a good father who listens to her and is interested in her without giving her advice all the time as her mother does. This seems to be a better "triangulation". From a psychological point of view, the term triangulation is a necessary aspect of child development when a third person intervenes in a two-party relationship. This enables the child to acquire new cognitive capacity.

The idea of triangulation was first put forwards by the Swiss psychiatrist Dr Ernest L. Abelin with particular focus on "early triangulation", whereby there are changes in psychoanalytic object relations theory and parent-child relationships when the child reaches the age of about 18 months. The mother is seen as the early caregiver having what could be described as a mutually stimulating relationship with the child, and the father, attracting and introducing the child to the world beyond this relationship, is therefore acting as the third party. This development of Mrs. X can be better identified later on when the patient has been condemned by her boss because of some mistakes in her work and she could cope with him because she had become more independent. But I think Mrs. X has several reasons to buy the house with her boyfriend. She is trying to give her daughter and herself a home and a feeling of a stable family. In addition to that, she is trying to keep her daughter at home because she wants to control her daughter, who is anorexic. Besides that, she avoids staying alone with her boyfriend if her daughter is still at home. Then she has repeatedly spoken about her coming to Germany when she was 13. She explained to me in that context that she had great language difficulties in school because she had not spoken German before; nevertheless, she made great progress at the end of the school year even though she did not achieve the high school certificate. She spoke in great detail and repeatedly about that period of her life. That means she wants it to be seen that she managed to deal successfully with that big problem and she is very proud of that. She said: "I had little confidence in myself to pass it!" Her dream job was to become a physiotherapist which she trained for; but she was very disappointed by this vocational course in Germany. She explained to me that that course in her country is offered only at a university and lasts for 5 years. In Germany, she had a few lectures, and the course lasts only for 3 years and she mainly had to work very hard in the hospital. Then she told me in the next session: "In the last session, we spoke about anger! Because of that I have had intense dreams". Here's the dream: My parents told me they wanted to go back to their country but they did not do that. Mrs. X had the feeling her parents had betrayed her. She expressed her anger against them. After that, she told me that she felt very relaxed and had been less tired. That means the therapy efforts helped her become more tolerant of and less threatened by her rage against her parents. Mrs. X has explored the origins of her anger in the therapy and realized the distortions in perception these often cause. She understood all that and because of that, she added then that she could not express her anger against her divorced husband. That means she has now a better feeling about her anger against significant others. Mrs. X is mainly concerned in that part of the therapy on her experiences with her migration to Germany and their consequences until today. She has described different forms of somatization, mainly a pressure in the middle of her belly at the solar plexus. If she then tried to relax, she would tremble, she told me. In that case, she felt detached from her emotions. Besides that, she has very often had dreams about that subject. She is repeatedly expressing her shock because she came and could not understand anything and had to go to school in Germany. She sees people from her country in her dreams who are deformed. For example, she sees some people from her country in Germany. They have leprosy, causing a lot of disabilities, and their hands are deformed and have

tattoos on their skin. She does not know these people because they are strange looking. They speak her first language. These dreams show the patient has been believing she is deformed and has leprosy symbolically because she is away from her
country. Mrs. X was able to interpret this dream in that way. Here is also one of her
dreams. She dreamed she has moved and been living faraway, and her grandmother
is also there, her great-grandmother and her boyfriend too. Her grandmother has
been living in a very beautiful residential home for the elderly. She commented
about that dream that her grandmother and her great-grandmother looked after her
when she was a child because her mother was working. Mrs. X has missed her
grandmother until today. She remembered she had no chance to say good bye to her
grandmother because she believed she was going to Germany only on holidays and
she would be seeing her again when she came back. When she actually came to
Germany, she was then informed she would be in Germany forever! This was a
shock to her and she could not grieve about the separation from her grandmother.
She explained to me that she was detached from her roots in that way. I as a therapist
am trying to activate her feelings. Thus, I ask her: "If you could now speak with
your grandmother and you could see your grandmother, what would you tell her?
She answers: "Do not emigrate! Thank you for looking after me!" She is obviously
trying to avoid emotions. I mention: "I do not think you are speaking with your
grandmother now!" She agrees with me and tells me with some tears in her eyes that
she could not speak with her grandmother now. She will fly the following week with
her mother to her country and she would try to speak with her there. After that, she
says she feels a warm pleasant feeling in her body, which means she expresses her
emotions again through her body. As you know, we call that somatization. She experiences that as an improvement. She says: "I am way ahead compared to last year! I
have the feeling that the therapy helps me!" At that time of the therapy, I would like
to mention that Mrs. X has recently followed a course of lectures about bookkeep-
ing, but she recognizes due to the therapy that she is having a really hard time now
(great pressure at work, problems with her daughter, the new house). From that
point of view, she decided to follow the lessons of the course but did not take part in
the final test. She decided she would do that later on when she has less stress. Apart
from that, she has got problems at work. The company where she worked was run-
ning the risk of becoming insolvent soon. Because of that, Mrs. X has been told she
needs to change her job in the company. She does not want that. She has found a
new job in her field and she is now negotiating with her new boss so that she can
continue the therapy. These vignettes demonstrate how she could come to acknowledge what puts her under great pressure and what is better for her health. She understands that she tends to have excessive expectations of herself. Through the therapy,
she tends to have more realistic ego ideal based on her real reasonable abilities. In
the further course of the therapy, Mrs. X focuses on her relationship with her daughter. Here she admits to herself for the first time, without feeling guilty, that when her
daughter was a child, she preferred to go to work rather than reduce her job in order
to be more available for her daughter. She controls the important others in identification with her mother and cannot let go. For example, during the coronavirus crisis, she puts her daughter, who was in another town at the time, under pressure to

come back and stay with her. Under the influence of her intense need to identify with her mother, she tends to control her daughter, and she is tense and suffers from muscle tension, especially in the back. I interpret her behaviour towards her daughter as having parallels with her mother's behaviour towards her. Mrs. X does not accept this interpretation; instead, she explains that her daughter cannot manage alone; she needs help because she is anorexic; thus, Mrs. X would like to put her daughter in a clinic. And she asks me if I could write an admission. I ask Mrs. X what her daughter wants herself. She is aware that her daughter is very ambivalent about therapy. Her daughter tries to analyse herself, but cannot free herself from problems. Thus, she noticed that her daughter was suffering greatly from this, which in turn was a great burden to her. Obviously, her daughter sends signals in the sense of a call for help, which makes it difficult for her to let go. She will change the shape of her relationship with her daughter, especially if she herself develops a better feeling of autonomy, which is the aim of the therapy. It remains to be seen whether she succeeds in this in the further course of therapy. So far, she definitely feels freer, more alive, and more driven. She has made herself aware that she has a very close relationship with her parents and tries to distance herself more from her mother or her parents. She has also become more aware of her perfectionism and that she often overtaxes herself against this background. In this sense, she begins to relativize her perfectionist demands on herself.

References

Arbeitskreis, O. P. D. (2006). *Operationalisierte Psychodynamische Diagnostik OPD-2. Das Manual für Diagnostik und Therapieplanung*. Bern: Huber.

Arieti, S., & Bemporad, J. R. (1980). The psychological organization of depression. *The American Journal of Psychiatry, 137*(11), 1360–1365.

Beck, A. T. (1983). Cognitive therapy of depression. New perspectives. In P. J. Clayton & J. M. Barrett (Eds.), *Treatment of depression: Old controversies and new approaches* (pp. 265–290). New York, NY: Raven.

Beutel, M. E., Wiltink, J., Hafner, C., Reiner, I., Bleichner, F., & Blatt, S. (2004). Abhängigkeit und Selbstkritik als psychologische Dimensionen der Depression-Validierung der deutschsprachigen Version des Depressive Experience Questionnaire (DEQ). *Zeitschrift für Klinische Psychologie, Psychiatrie und Psychotherapie, 1*, 1–14.

Bibring, E. (1952). Das problem der depression. *Psyche, 6*(2), 81–101.

Blatt, S. J. (1998). Contributions of psychoanalysis to the understanding and treatment of depression. *Journal of the American Psychoanalytic Association, 46*(3), 723–752.

Blatt, S. J. (2004). *Experiences of depression: Theoretical clinical and research perspectives*. Washington, DC: American Psychological Association.

Blatt, S. J. (2005). A dialectic model of personality development and psychopathology: Recent contributions to understanding and treating depression. In J. Corveleyn, P. Luyten, & S. J. Blatt (Eds.), *The theory and treatment of depression: Towards a dynamic interactionism model* (pp. 137–162). Hillsdale, NJ: Lawrence Erlbaum Associates.

Blatt, S. J., & Blass, R. B. (1996). Relatedness and self-definition: A dialectic model of personality development. In G. G. Noam & K. W. Fischer (Eds.), *Development and vulnerabilities on close relationships* (pp. 309–338). Hillsdale, NJ: Lawrence Erlbaum Associates.

Blatt, S. J., D'Afflitti, J. P., & Quinlan, D. M. (1976). Experiences of depression in normal young adults. *Journal of Abnormal Psychology, 85*(4), 383.

Blatt, S. J., Luyten, P., & Corveleyn, J. (2005). Zur Entwicklung eines dynamischen Interaktionsmodells der Depression und ihrer Behandlung. *Psyche, 59*(9–10), 864–891.

Blatt, S. J., & Maroudas, C. (1992). Convergences among psychoanalytic and cognitive-behavioral theories of depression. *Psychoanalytic Psychology, 9*(2), 157–190.

Cohen, M. B., Blake, C. M., Grace, B., Cohen, R. A., Fromm-Reichmann, F., & Weigert, E. V. (1954). An intensive study of twelve cases of manic-depressive psychosis. *Psychiatry, 17*(2), 103–137.

Enns, M. W., Cox, B. J., & Clara, I. (2002). Adaptive and maladaptive perfectionism: Developmental origins and association with depression proneness. *Personality and Individual Differences, 33*(6), 921–935.

Freud, S. (1916–1917). *Trauer und Melacholie. Gesammelte Werke Band X.* London: Imago Publishing Co., Ltd..

Luyten, P. (2002). *Normbesef en depressie: Aanzet tot een integraitef theoratisch kader en een empirisch onderzoek aan de hand van de depressietheorie van S. J. Blatt.* Unpublished doctoral dissertation, University Leuven, Belgium.

Reis, S., & Grenyer, B. F. (2002). Pathways to anaclitic and introjective depression. *Psychology and Psychotherapy: Theory, Research and Practice, 75*(4), 445–459.

Shahar, G., & Mayes, L. C. (2017). Sidney Blatt's psychoanalytic legacy: An introduction. *Journal of the American Psychoanalytic Association, 65*(3), 453–456.

Chapter 7
The LAC Study: Chronic Depression and Relationship to Childhood Trauma

Marianne Leuzinger-Bohleber

Contents

7.1   Introduction[1]

In recent decades, depression has increased to such an extent that, according to WHO estimates, it becomes the second most widespread disease worldwide in 2020 (see, e.g., Bromet et al., 2011; Murphy & Byrne, 2012; Vandeleur et al., 2017; WHO, 2013/2017). Twenty percent to 33% of individuals with a depressive disorder develop a chronic course (Murphy & Byrne, 2012; Spijker, van Straten, Bockting, Meeuwissen, & van Balkom, 2013; Steinert, Hofmann, Kruse, & Leichsenring, 2014). Subjects with chronic depression are the most severely affected among

---

[1]This chapter is based on former publications (e.g., Leuzinger-Bohleber, 2005; Leuzinger-Bohleber, Hautzinger, et al., 2019; Leuzinger-Bohleber, Kallenbach, et al., 2020; Leuzinger-Bohleber, Kaufhold, et al., 2019; Leuzinger-Bohleber, Solms, & Arnold, 2020).

M. Leuzinger-Bohleber (✉)
Universitymedicine Mainz, Mainz, Germany
e-mail: mleuzing@uni-mainz.de

© Springer Nature Switzerland AG 2021   81
C. Charis, G. Panayiotou (eds.), *Depression Conceptualization and Treatment*,
https://doi.org/10.1007/978-3-030-68932-2_7

depressive patients, with greater severity of depression, more frequent depressive episodes, higher rates of other psychiatric and physical comorbidities (Hung, Liu, & Yang, 2019; Klein, Shankman, & Rose, 2006; Murphy & Byrne, 2012; Vandeleur et al., 2017), and a longer duration of pharmacotherapy and a lower remission rate (Hung et al., 2019). Chronic depression is also associated with enormous suffering for those affected and their families and enormous direct and indirect health costs.

For a long time, depression was considered a disorder with a relatively good treatment prognosis, but this has changed in recent decades. Results from epidemiological research showed that depression is often a recurrent disorder with a high relapse rate and becomes chronic. Fifty percent of the depressed patients suffer a relapse after the first depressive episode, 70% after the second episode, and 90% after the third episode. In addition, pharmacological and short psychotherapeutic cognitive-behavioral as well as short psychotherapeutic treatment approaches have proved to be far less successful than hoped: 50% of all depressed patients have a relapse after any form of short psychotherapy (see Blatt & Zuroff, 2005). Twenty percent to 30% of all depressed patients do not respond positively to drugs at all (see, e.g., Corveleyn, Luyten, Blatt, & Lens-Gielis, 2013; Huhn et al., 2014; Trivedi, Nieuwsma, & Williams, 2011). Of those with a positive response, one third has a relapse within 1 year, 75% within 5 years (see also Cuipers, Huibers, & Furukawa, 2017; Steinert et al., 2014). For these patients, long-term psychoanalytic therapies or psychoanalyses may offer an alternative (see Leichsenring, 2008; Leichsenring & Rabung, 2011; Leuzinger-Bohleber, Hautzinger, et al., 2019; Leuzinger-Bohleber, Kaufhold, et al., 2019). In the representative DPV outcome study, e.g., around 80% of all the 402 former psychoanalyses patients or patients of long-term psychoanalytic therapies has shown sustained improvements in their psychopathological symptoms as well as in their object relations, professional quality, and life quality. Among them, there were 27% who had been diagnosed as depressed mostly in combination with some personality disorders. To mention just one of the unexpected results of the study: 62% of the patients had been severely traumatized children of the Second World War (cf. Leuzinger-Bohleber, Stuhr, Rüger, & Beutel, 2003).

Although depression can be regarded as one of the psychoanalytically best investigated disorders, the differentiation between its various forms is by no means easy and not yet sufficiently understood. The older definition focused on psychogenic, endogenic, and somatogenic depression, and then DSM-IV and ICD-10 started from the descriptive-symptomatic level and arrived at dimensionally different disorders (major depression, dysthymia, etc.). Without excluding the biological factors, in a psychodynamic understanding of depression, the forms are not fanned out categorically or dimensionally (see, e.g., Hill, 2009). Thus, as Sidney Blatt (2004) suggests, the different forms of depression can be located on a continuum ranging from the dysphoric mood of microdepression to severe depression.

According to Bohleber (2005, 2010), in *social sciences, depression has advanced to a signature of our time*, in which traditional structures and clear behavioral expectations have largely dissolved. Phenomena of delimitation and the enormous increase of individuums choices of life perspectives result in a loss of social security and make one's own identity the lifelong project of the individual. In his study, the

French sociologist Alain Ehrenberg (2016) declares the exhausted self to be the disease of contemporary society, whose behavioral norms are no longer based on guilt and discipline, but mainly on responsibility and initiative. The late bourgeois individual seems to be replaced by an individual who has the idea that "everything is possible" and is marked by the fear for his self-realization, which can easily increase to the feeling of exhaustion. The pressure for individualization is reflected in feelings of failure, shame, and insufficiency and finally in depressive symptoms. For Ehrenberg, if neurosis is the illness of the individual torn apart by the conflict between what is allowed and what is forbidden, depression is the illness of the individual inhibited and exhausted by the tension between what is possible and what is impossible. Depression thus becomes a tragedy of inadequacy (for the role of social and cultural factors in depression: see also Jimenez, 2019).

Such epistemological-clinical data and social-scientific analyses also challenge psychoanalysis to re-examine the issue of depression and evaluate the state of its research. In the meantime, the outcomes of psychoanalytic *short-term therapies* according to evidence-based medicine criteria have been confirmed by many studies (see, e.g., Abbass, Kisely, & Kroenke, 2009; De Maat et al., 2013; Driessen et al., 2010; Fonagy, 2015; Kächele & Thomä, 2000; Shedler, 2010, 2015). Liliengren (2019) has collected 272 RCT studies in this field until now (see also the third edition of the Open Door Review, Leuzinger-Bohleber, Arnold, & Kaechele, 2015/2019). In contrast, still only a few studies are available on the effects of long-term psychotherapies and psychoanalyses (see, e.g., Blomberg, 2001; Fonagy, Luyten, & Allison, 2015; Fonagy, Rost, et al., 2015; Grande et al., 2009; Huber & Klug, 2016; Knekt et al., 2011; Leichsenring, 2008; Leichsenring & Rabung, 2011). Therefore, in 2005, a multicenter research group of psychoanalysts and cognitive behaviorists decided to initiate a comparative psychotherapy study on the outcomes of cognitive-behavioral and psychoanalytic long-term treatments, the so-called *LAC study*. We conceptualized the study in close collaboration with the research group of Phil Richardson, Peter Fonagy, and David Taylor, who also—at that time—planned a study on the outcome of psychoanalytic long-term psychotherapies in difficult-to-treat depression, the so-called *Tavistock Depression Study*. We used a number of identical measuring instruments to compare the data from the two studies. Close collaboration was also established on the psychoanalytic conceptualization of depression. David Taylor had just written first versions of the Tavistock Treatment Manual for the treatment of difficult-to-treat, depressed patients. He agreed to train the psychoanalytic study therapists of the LAC study, a prerequisite for us to include psychoanalysts of various psychoanalytical orientations as study therapists.[2]

---

[2] Already in the LAC study, we assumed that we wanted to investigate – in the sense of a naturalistic study – psychoanalytic long-term treatments, as they are really carried out in the private offices in Germany, financed by the health insurance companies. Therefore, we assumed a thorough psychoanalytic training of the therapists and required at least 3 years of experience after completion of their trainings. The additional training in David Taylor's manual then built on this "foundation of psychoanalytic knowledge" and sensitized the study therapists to specific challenges in the treatment technique of this difficult-to-treat group of patients.

In the meantime, both the results of the Tavistock study (Fonagy, Luyten, & Allison, 2015; Fonagy, Rost, et al., 2015) and the LAC study (Leuzinger-Bohleber, Hautzinger, et al., 2019; Leuzinger-Bohleber, Kaufhold, et al., 2019) have been published.[3] These and several other studies show the positive outcomes of long-term psychoanalytic therapies for depressed patients (see Sect. 7.2).[4] The main focus of this chapter is an unexpected finding of the LAC study: around 80% of the chronic depressed patients had suffered from severe childhood trauma. We are summarizing these findings in Sect. 7.3 which have a high relevance for the transmission of trauma and depression to the next generation, as will be discussed in Sect. 7.4. An extensive case example will illustrate our empirical findings.

7.2   The LAC Study (*L*angzeitbehandlungen *c*hronisch Depressiver): A Randomized Controlled Study Comparing the Outcomes of Long-Term Psychoanalytical and Cognitive-Behavioral Psychotherapies with Chronic Depressed Patients

The curiosity to find out more about the factors involved in psychoanalytic treatment compared to long-term CBT, the threat of social denial of psychoanalysis, but also the interest of some CBT researchers in getting longer treatments financed by the health insurance funds were the reasons why an interdisciplinary research group decided in 2005 to initiate a multicenter study on the outcome of cognitive and psychoanalytic long-term treatment in chronic depressive patients, the LAC study (project chairs: M. Leuzinger-Bohleber, M. Hautzinger, M. Beutel, G. Fiedler, W. Keller). The planning and implementation of the LAC study took place against the background of many controversial discussions (see, e.g., Leuzinger-Bohleber,

---

It is well-known that for the acceptance of outcome studies in times of evidence-based medicine, it is necessary to use treatment manuals. This also applies to psychoanalytic long-term treatments. However, as we have discussed in various papers, these manuals have a different character from manuals for short-term psychoanalytic therapies. Especially, the group of chronically depressed patients requires a lot of creativity, originality, and flexibility from the psychoanalyst to reach the patient emotionally, to initiate a therapeutic process at all, as well as to work through the idiosyncratic unconscious conflicts and fantasies of the chronically depressed in the transference relationship. Nevertheless, the creative psychoanalyst will need to follow specific psychoanalytic treatment techniques that are described in a "manual."

[3] We thank David Taylor. Peter Fonagy, and Phil Richardson, who sadly died much too early, for their continuous support of the LAC study. We also thank all the patients, colleagues, and scientists who have been evolved in the LAC study as well as the DGPT, the DPV, the IPA, and Dr. von der Tann for the generous financial support of the study.

[4] Of course, we still need more studies on the outcomes of psychoanalytical long-term therapies. Therefore, we are realizing of a replication study of the LAC study at the moment: the *Multi-Level Outcome Study of Psychoanalyses of Chronically Depressed Patients with Early Trauma (MODE)*.

Solms, & Arnold, 2020). For example, the research group opted for a design that combines a naturalistic study with an experimental one. In contrast to many studies of comparative psychotherapy research, in which for methodical and pragmatic reasons, trained students or study therapists treated persons with precisely defined symptoms (often students) according to a manualized therapy method, in the LAC study, chronically depressive patients, as they are treated in private practices of psychotherapists in Germany today, were seen by experienced therapists in long-term psychotherapies. We expected that many of them had already undergone several shorter therapies with only limited success, or even negative results, and therefore had a preference for a certain therapeutic procedure. They would therefore not be willing to be randomized for long-term treatment. Therefore, in the LAC study, they could choose between the two therapies, cognitive-behavioral therapy (CBT) and psychoanalytic long-term therapy (PAT). If they did not have a clear preference and were willing to do so, they were randomized. psychoanalytic therapy (PAT).

In 2005, PAT and CBT had been the only forms of psychotherapy which—due to enough empirical studies of their efficiency—had been supported by the insurance companies in Germany. These treatments had been summarized here shortly (see Tables 7.1 and 7.2).

This basic CBT for depression could be extended for chronic depressed patients by additional intervention elements (e.g., situational analysis, skill training, self-disclosure). All study CBT therapists were well trained and state licensed. They saw patients regularly, either in their own private practice or as therapists in cooperating outpatient units. Furthermore, they all participated in an initiating workshop about CBT of chronic depression and were supervised throughout the study. Supervision was offered at each site by experienced senior CBT therapists. At each site, workshops were offered regularly (one per year) to the study therapists. Each therapy session has been taped, and a selection of tapes of each therapy have been rated to control for adherence to cognitive-behavioral therapy and for therapists' competence.

Randomization of the patients, precisely described inclusion criteria, blind raters, reliable measuring instruments, manualized therapy procedures checked for their adherence, as well as the exact description of the samples, dropouts and applied statistical procedures, etc. belong to the criteria of the so-called evidence-based medicine. These criteria must be met in order for the studies to be recognized both in the world of psychotherapy research and in healthcare systems. Therefore, the research group of the LAC study tried to meet all these criteria.

In addition, the well-known epistemological and methodological concerns of the psychoanalytic community were taken seriously, and a multi-perspective approach to the therapeutic outcome of these "difficult-to-treat" patients was chosen. Thus, in the second main publication of the LAC study, one aspect of this complex problem was presented for discussion as an example: in the world of evidence-based medicine, it is well-known that almost exclusively symptom changes are regarded as a success for psychotherapies, whereas psychodynamically, changes in the inner

Table 7.1 Psychoanalytic psychotherapy

Psychoanalytic psychotherapy is well developed for severely and chronically depressed patients with comorbidity (see, e.g., Leuzinger-Bohleber, 2015b; Taylor, 2010). Psychoanalytic authors have considered depression in the context of developmental processes, particularly pathological processes determined by unconscious fantasies and conflicts concerning (a) a differentiated, integrated, and realistic basic feeling of self and identity; (b) the ability to engage in satisfying reciprocal interpersonal relationships; and (c) the ability to unfold one's own creativity in work, developmental tasks matching the patient's lifecycle, and satisfying management of everyday life situations. Discovering the unconscious determining factors due to failures in the development (archaic unconscious fantasies stimulated by traumatization, pathological relationships, burdened life situations, etc.) and working through idiosyncratic unconscious fantasies and conflicts due to developmental deficits and traumatization in the "here and now" of the therapeutic relationship is seen as indispensable for a long-lasting change of depressive symptoms. Thus, different forms of depression are not understood as clearly distinct entities due to specific genetic or neurobiological factors, but as products of complex interactions between genetic vulnerabilities and experiences in early relationships leading to pathological fantasies, developments, and adaptations. They constitute maladaptive attempts of the individual to cope with severe and lasting disruptions of his normal development. All psychoanalytic study therapists of the LAC study were trained in the Tavistock manual for treating chronic depressed patients in different workshops. This manual details psychoanalytic techniques to be applied with this group of patients, illustrated by clinical "anchor examples." Pretested in a British trial with chronically depressed patients, it specifies a therapeutic approach, including establishing emotional contact, receptivity, and openness and identification of fears, activity, and work in the "here and now" and in transference. A psychodynamic model of the evolvement of chronic depression provides a background of specific interventions. Psychoanalysts have had at least 3 years of clinical practice, participated in regular supervision groups, and were asked to record at least 40 therapy sessions, to permit independent control for adherence and competence

Table 7.2 Cognitive-behavioral therapy

Cognitive-behavioral therapy for depression followed a widely used and well-accepted CBT manual. Nearly all licensed behavioral therapists are familiar with this manual and material and have received formal training in using the manual. In general, CBT with depressed patients follows five phases within 25–45 sessions: *Phase 1*, development, biographical information, problem analysis, goals, psycho-education, rationale for treatment, explanation of intervention steps; *Phase 2*, behavior-oriented interventions, activation, increasing pleasant activities, balance of negative and positive activities, situation analysis, structuring day and week; *Phase 3*, cognitive interventions, thought control, focus on automatic thoughts and alternatives, influence basic assumptions and schemata; *Phase 4*, skill training, social skills, problem-solving skills, communication skills, role-play, stress management, etc.; *Phase 5*, maintenance, prepare for crisis and beginning depression, relapse prevention, transfer into everyday life

world of objects, so-called structural changes, characterize successful psychotherapies, because the goal of psychoanalytic treatments goes far beyond symptom
changes and, as Freud postulated, is described as the ability to love, to work, and to
enjoy life (cf., e.g., Leuzinger-Bohleber, Hautzinger, et al., 2019; Leuzinger-
Bohleber, Kaufhold, et al., 2019). Therefore, symptomatic and structural changes
were compared and contrasted in the LAC study (cf. Kaufhold et al., 2019).

In the meantime, the *Canadian Journal of Psychiatry* (Leuzinger-Bohleber, Hautzinger, et al., 2019) has published the main results concerning symptomatic changes. In a second article in the *International Journal of Psychoanalysis*, the results of symptomatic and structural changes were compared (Kaufhold et al., 2019; Leuzinger-Bohleber, Kaufhold, et al., 2019). In addition, the modifications of the two English articles with comments by Peter Fonagy (psychoanalyst) and John Clarkin (behavioral therapist) were made available to a German readership in a special issue of *PSYCHE* in February 2019.

Therefore, in this chapter, I can refer to the publications already published and limit myself to a summary of the methodological approach and the results both with regard to the symptom and the structural change.

7.3 Summary of the Design and the Main Results of the LAC Study

The LAC depression study is the first to compare the long-term effectiveness of cognitive-behavioral therapy (CBT) and psychoanalytic therapy (PAT) of chronic depressed patients with a study design that investigates the influence of treatment preference in contrast to randomized assignment. The aim of the study is to compare those two treatments according to their short-term and long-term effects on different outcome variables regarding depressive symptoms, remission rates, the level of psychosocial outcome variables, etc. The authors hypothesize that both treatments lead to symptomatic improvements, whereas PAT starts more slowly than CBT but achieves more stable effects (measured by the primary outcome instruments, BDI, and QIDS-C) (Beutel et al., 2012). Figure 7.1 shows the scope and sequence of assessments.[5]

We have published the CONSORT diagram with detailed analyses of the recruitment of the patients, the reasons for being excluded from the study, and how many of the patients remained in the study (see Leuzinger-Bohleber, Hautzinger, et al., 2019). A total of 554 patients were interviewed. Of those, 252 patients were included in the study. Study patients were followed for 3 years receiving preferred or randomly assigned treatment. Typical for a naturalistic treatment setting, treatment ended upon mutual agreement of therapist and patient. Based on the total sample of 252 study patients, at least one outcome criterion (BDI or QIDS) was available (indicating that the patients still were included in the study) for 73.4% after 1 year,

---

[5] We decided to publish the first outcome paper after 3 years after beginning of treatment for different reasons: the research group of the LAC study had been working already for 15 years. Therefore, it was absolutely necessary to have the main outcome results now published. This makes it possible for the younger members of the research group to publish further results, e.g., in the frame of their doctoral theses, etc. – this means that some few psychoanalytic treatments are still ongoing and that not all patients have been investigated 5 years after the beginning of treatment.

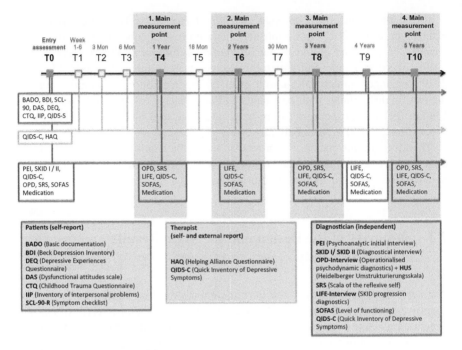

Fig. 7.1 Data assessment: LAC study

63.9% after 2 years, and 65.5% after 3 years. Compared to other studies, this is a good response rate (see, e.g., Fonagy, Luyten, & Allison, 2015; Fonagy, Rost, et al., 2015).[6]

The baseline demographic and clinical characteristics of all study subjects have been published in detail (see Leuzinger-Bohleber, Hautzinger, et al., 2019). Patients suffered from chronic depression of high current symptom severity (BDI 32.1 points; QIDS-C 14.3 points). These scores corresponded to percent rank above 75 in large samples of depressed patients. The majority had long sick leaves from work due to their depression during the past year. More than 70% had had previous psychotherapies, some even four and more treatments. More than one third of our sample had been admitted to inpatient psychotherapy. Thirty-six percent were on antidepressant medication. According to DSM-IV, 58.3% fulfilled MDE criteria of a major depression (MDE), 12.3% suffered of dysthymia, and 29.4% were diagnosed with double depression. It proved to be much more difficult to recruit patients who were willing to be randomized than originally expected. In spite of enormous efforts, only 88 subjects could be randomly assigned to one of the two psychotherapies, while 164 subjects were assigned according to their treatment preference.

---

[6] The homogeneity of the sample was tested by the methodological center (see Leuzinger-Bohleber, Kallenbach, et al., 2020; Leuzinger-Bohleber, Solms, & Arnold, 2020).

Treatment effects by self-report (BDI) and blinded expert rating (QIDS-C) over the course of 3 years were analyzed using linear mixed models. Thus, we were able to include $N = 252$ patients into our study. The dependent variables were the BDI and QIDS-C scores of the patients 1, 2, and 3 years after treatment starts (time points T4, T6, T8). Time points of observation and the four treatment groups of the patient (CBT, PAT, randomized, preference) were included as independent variables. Intake of medication was controlled based on the baseline findings.

7.4   Findings on Symptomatic Changes in Long-Term Psychotherapies

Both psychotherapies achieved a significant reduction of symptoms in these patients, who were often had been ill for a long time. After only 1 year, the BDI score of 32.1 points decreased by 12.1 points, and after 3 years, by as much as 17.2 points (self-assessment by patients). The effect sizes were very high: $d = 1.17$ after 1 year and $d = 1.83$ after 3 years. Analogous results were shown in the assessments of the independent blinded raters with regard to the form of treatment. The QIDS-C score decreased from 14.1 to 7.1 in the first year and further to 7.0 in 3 years after the start of treatment. The effect sizes were also very high: they increased from $d = 1.56$ after 1 year to $d = 2.08$ after 3 years after the start of treatment. The remission rates achieved are better than in other studies: 39% of patients showed full remission after only 1 year, and 61% after 3 years of treatment. Chronically depressive patients therefore benefit from long-term psychotherapy.

Psychoanalytic as well as cognitive-behavioral therapy thus achieved sustained improvements of depressive symptoms of chronic depressed patients, but of course, critical evaluators will argue that psychoanalysis needs more sessions for achieving this symptomatic improvement.[7] Over the 3 years, PAT had a total of 234 sessions on average, while CBT had only on average a total of 57 sessions during the study period. PAT patients were in treatment for up to 36 months, while last CBT patients ended treatment after 15 months.

In the discussion of our first outcome paper focusing on symptomatic changes, we have argued as follows:

---

[7] We tried to keep the dose of the treatments comparable during the first year—afterward the treatments should continue according to the needs of the patients and the conceptualization of the treatments by the therapists (e.g., CBT followed the guidelines of a so-called relapse prevention therapy). According to the study protocol, PAT should not offer more than 80 sessions, CBT not less than 60 sessions during the first year of treatment. Our data showed that the therapists followed more their naturalistic practices than the study protocol: PAT had a mean of 80.4 sessions (SD 27.8) during the first year of treatment, while CBT had only a mean of 32.5 (SD 9.0) therapy sessions.

PAT and CBT offered different intensities and durations of treatment due to their divergent theoretical conceptualizations of chronic depression and of the treatment process (…). In order to determine if improvements were due to common factors such as contact over time with the therapist or specific factors associated with each treatment modality (e.g., structural change in PAT) we will identify moderator and mediator variables for successful outcome of PAT, respectively CBT. We have included a comprehensive set of secondary outcome criteria such as structural change, social adaptation, quality of social relationships and therapeutic alliance to be used in such analyses (…). Future analyses will also scrutinize sub-groups of chronically depressed patients who improved more in PAT or in CBT and how they differ from patients with less favorable outcomes. This will offer important insights into the relevant question, which chronically depressed patients need which kind and amount of treatment (…). Analyses of direct and indirect costs of these treatments will also be done in future publications. (Leuzinger-Bohleber, Hautzinger, et al., 2019, p. 8)

Therefore, several additional analyses of the data of the LAC study are in progress and will be published soon. As already mentioned: one paper concerning the second outcome measures, investigating one further dimension of psychic transformations, the so-called structural changes in both treatments, has already been published and is considered as the second main outcome paper of this large study (Kaufhold et al., 2019; Leuzinger-Bohleber, Hautzinger, et al., 2019). In this context, we can only summarize the main findings:

7.5 Findings on Structural Changes in Long-Term Treatments

Following the psychoanalytical conceptualization of depression, chronic depressed patients suffer from pathological self- and object representations connected to unbearable emotions (despair, helplessness, hopelessness) and chronic dissociative states of the mind. Modifying structural deficits in the self-object representations takes time and an intensive working through in the professional "corrective" emotional relationship to the psychotherapist. These sustaining psychic transformations or so called structural changes are described in detail in other publications (Kaufhold et al., 2019; Leuzinger-Bohleber, Hautzinger, et al., 2019; Leuzinger-Bohleber, Kaufhold, et al., 2019). Thus, structural changes have been one of the central secondary outcome measures. We have measured them by the Operationalized Psychodynamic Diagnostics (OPD) and the Heidelberg Structural Change Scale (HSCS) (vgl. Rudolf et al., 2012, detailed description in Kaufhold et al., 2019; Leuzinger-Bohleber, Hautzinger, et al., 2019; Leuzinger-Bohleber, Solms, & Arnold, 2020). With these instruments, the increasing awareness of patients for their psychodynamically significant unconscious fantasies and conflicts was examined, which is regarded as an important prerequisite for structural changes in the sense of HSCS. Even if it is not yet possible to record lasting changes in therapy after 3 years after the beginning of treatment, the results indicate differences between patients in psychoanalytic and long-term behavioral therapy already at this time point.

The intrapsychic conflicts or structural deficits assessed at the beginning of treatment did not differ between CBT and PAT. The frequencies of the focuses identified by the raters blinded to the treatment condition in both treatment groups corresponded to psychodynamic conceptualizations of chronically depressed patients (cf., e.g., Leuzinger-Bohleber, 2015b): problems in connection with the structural dimensions of "self-regulation," "internal communication," and the conflict focus of "care versus self-sufficiency." According to the HSCS thesis, changes in the conscious perception of these focuses can lead to sustaining psychological transformations in depressive patients in the sense of structural changes. One year after the start of treatment, the proportions of structural changes between PAT (26%) and CBT (24%) were only insignificantly different. After 3 years, at 60%, more patients in PAT met the criteria for a structural change in comparison to CBT (36%)—analogous to the objective in these treatments. In the control of baseline HSCS, sex and age, the treatment arm remained a highly significant predictor of structural changes; in general, the therapy procedure was able to predict the structural changes. In PAT, these changes were significantly more frequent than in CBT 3 years after the start of treatment. Further analyses showed that the structural changes defined by OPD/HSCS are also a predictor of symptomatic changes. As the interaction of therapy formed and structural change showed, after 3 years, there was a stronger correlation between structural changes and reduction of depressive symptoms in PAT than in CBT.

Thus, structural change, defined by increasing awareness of psychodynamically relevant unconscious intrapsychic conflicts and deficits in mental structure, proved to be particularly relevant for long-term psychoanalytic psychotherapies. In line with the model of Lane, Ryan, Nadel, and Greenberg (2015), a structural change requires a high emotional intensity in the therapeutic relationship and takes time. The psychoanalytic technique of working intensively with patients in the therapeutic relationship over a long period of time can create an extraordinary opportunity to activate emotions and associated "embodied memories" of unconscious, early traumatic experiences. They learn to endure them in the therapeutic relationship and—thanks to the analyst's containment and holding function—to relive them emotionally in their hitherto unbearable intensity. This makes these memories accessible to a common understanding. These activations and the therapeutic working through make it possible to observe in detail the specific influence of traumatic experiences on current conflicts and emotional experiences in transmission with an emotional intensity and liveliness that, according to Lane et al. (2015), is difficult to achieve with other psychotherapeutic methods.[8] As illustrated in a detailed case study (Leuzinger-Bohleber, Hautzinger, et al., 2019, p. 113 ff.), traumatization and the unconscious fantasies stimulated by the traumatic loss could be integrated into a more mature self and identity, which were no longer unconsciously determined by past traumatization and associated fantasies and conflicts (cf., e.g., Bohleber &

---

[8] In the replication study of the LAC study, MODE, we are systematically investigating these hypotheses applying a broad range of psychological, psychoanalytical, and neurobiological measurements (see Peterson et al., 2019).

Leuzinger-Bohleber, 2016; Negele, Kaufhold, Kallenbach, & Leuzinger-Bohleber, 2015).

These are possible explanations as to why structural changes were observed more frequently in patients in PAT after 3 years of treatment than in the CBT group. We expect structural changes to continue to consolidate in the upcoming analysis of the LAC study data 5 years after treatment initiation. It is currently being examined whether these changes are associated with a reduction in incapacity to work, one of the sources of the enormous indirect health costs associated with chronic depression. Shedler (2010) summarized as follows: "Especially noteworthy is the recurring finding that the benefits of psychodynamic therapy not only endure but increase with time, a finding that has now emerged from at least five independent meta-analyses […]. In contrast, the benefits of other (non-psychodynamic) empirically supported therapies tend to decay overtime for the most common disorders" (p. 101 f).

From a cognitive-behavioral perspective, we need to understand by what mechanisms deeply ingrained maladaptive behavior patterns are influenced by less intensive intervention. The mechanism of change should be different between CBT and PAT or structural changes can be achieved by more confronting, active, focused interventions. We have assessed study patients with identical batteries of tests and interviews. This should make it possible to take a step closer to answer such questions.

Therefore, we hope to gain further insights through the ongoing detailed data analyses as to which of the chronically depressed patients are more likely to be treated with psychoanalytic long-term therapy and which with cognitive-behavioral long-term therapy. We owe this to these seriously ill people and their years of suffering: the times of horse racing between different psychotherapy schools and the associated fantasy of omnipotence, that one certain approach is suitable for every patient, are over.

7.6 Childhood Trauma and Depression: Some Psychoanalytical Considerations

As mentioned above, one of the unexpected results of the LAC study was the striking accumulation of early trauma in the sample of chronically depressed people. Alexa Negele (2015) has dedicated her doctoral thesis to this topic. Three hundred forty-nine chronically depressed patients who had been seen during the screening for the LAC depression study completed the Childhood Trauma Questionnaire, a self-report measure of traumatic experiences in childhood. Seventy-six percent of the depressed patients reported clinically significant histories of childhood trauma. Thirty-seven percent of the depressed patients reported multiple childhood traumatization. Experiences of multiple trauma also led to significantly more severe depressive symptoms. Stepwise multiple regression analysis suggested that childhood emotional abuse and sexual abuse were significantly associated with a vulnerability to chronic depression in adulthood. Clinical implications suggest a precise assessment of childhood trauma in chronically depressed patients with a focus on emotional abuse, sexual abuse, and multiple trauma.

Negele et al. (2015) summarize the findings: "Women reported significantly more frequent of childhood trauma in general and of emotional and sexual abuse in particular." McGrath, Keita, Stickland, and Russo (1993) pointed to the higher risk of victimization in women and estimated childhood abuse in women at 21.7–37%. Lampe's (2002) review on childhood trauma confirmed that women suffered more frequently from sexual abuse than men. Scher, Forde, McQuaid, and Stein (2004) showed that women were nearly twice as likely to report emotional abuse and were nearly four times as likely to report sexual abuse. Arnow, Blasely, Hunkeler, Lee, and Hayward (2012) examined the moderating role of gender on the association between childhood trauma and depression, yet found no gender differences. However, they also identified significantly more women than men reporting histories of emotional abuse and sexual abuse.

Furthermore, our results suggest a substantial influence of multiple childhood trauma on a chronic course of depression in adulthood. Thirty-seven percent of our patients reported a history of multiple childhood trauma; additionally, 18.1% achieved thresholds on at least two subscales. Also in line with other studies (e.g., Widom, DuMont, & Czaja, 2007), the patients reporting multiple childhood trauma showed greater symptom severity suggesting a dose-response relationship between childhood trauma and chronicity of depression. Co-occurrences of childhood trauma and its possible effects being synergistic or additive (Fischer & Riedesser, 2009; Teicher, Samson, Polcari, & Andersen, 2009) due to cumulative, sequential, simultaneous, and/or complex (Herman, 1992; van der Kolk, 2005) impacts may be specifically relevant in chronically depressed patients.

Though childhood abuse can be viewed as a relatively nonspecific risk factor for later psychopathology, specific contributions of certain types of childhood trauma to the vulnerability of different forms of psychopathology were repeatedly reported. Our results show that emotional abuse with 61% was reported most frequently. Additionally, 25% of the patients reported sexual abuse. Contrastingly, 15% emotional abuse and 12.6% sexual abuse were found in a representative German survey study on the prevalence of childhood trauma (Häuser, Schmutzer, Brähler, & Glaesmer, 2011). Regression analysis showed emotional abuse and sexual abuse to be specifically related to chronic depression. Yet, both types only accounted for a poor amount of variance (4–6%), hence providing solely limited explanatory power.

Stress childhood sexual abuse as a serious relational trauma and conceptualize childhood sexual abuse itself as multiple trauma (p. 303). Wetzel (1998), for example, found that 64.3% of sexually abused participants were at the same time physically abused. Molnar, Buka, and Kessler (2001) examined the relation between childhood sexual abuse and later psychopathology and reported significantly higher percentages of women and men with lifetime dysthymia (15.7% and 12.5%) and depression (39.3% and 30.3%) among those reporting of childhood sexual abuse.

Briere and Elliott (1994) link experiences of childhood sexual abuse to disruptions in the development of a sense of self again causing difficulties in relating to others. The study of Molnar et al. (2001) showed the highest odds ratios of rape by family members for PTSD. Unfortunately, the CTQ subscale for sexual abuse lacks information on perpetrators and the victims' relations to them, so conclusions on familial vs. nonfamilial sexual abuse cannot be drawn.

Experiences of emotional abuse characterize an atmosphere of being related to others. In this sense, depression can again be related to trauma as a "relational" term. Attachment theory (e.g., Bowlby, 1980), processes of identification and introjection, or the herein comprised loss of a sense of worth, well-being, or self-efficacy (...)[9] might explain its strong connection to a more chronic course of depression. It marks, as to the disruption of one's capacity to ascribe meaning in trauma, the loss of a basic sense of trust and an enduring shock of one's understanding of the outer and the inner world (Bohleber, 2010). In addition, emotionally abused children may attribute more negatively which may lead into the development of a more general negative attribution style again leading to depression (...).

For example, Gibb and Alloy (2006) investigated the potential of emotional abuse to change children's inferential styles in a sample of 140 children of parents with a depression history. They found that emotional abuse was significantly related to changes in children's inferential styles regarding consequences and self-characteristics.

Our findings suggest implications for clinical practice. Clinicians should precisely look for the presence of childhood trauma in chronically depressed patients being aware of its possible prognostic implications. Especially emotional abuse, sexual abuse and multiple traumatic experiences may lead to a more chronic course of depression. Nonetheless, a group of likewise severely depressed patients reporting histories of childhood trauma subthreshold as conceptualized within this study remained. This underlines that childhood trauma may only be one central pathway leading to chronic depression in adulthood (...). Depression summarizes a group of highly complex mental disorders that have to be diagnosed precisely and treated cautiously in consideration of its origins" (Negele et al., 2015, p.).

Fortunately, the long-term influence of trauma and depression is now increasingly discussed in the more recent psychoanalytical literature (overview in Bohleber, 2005, 2010). Hugo Bleichmar (1996, 2013) also mentions severe trauma in his frequently cited model as a possible path leading to depression (see Fig. 7.2).

In most cases, this refers to traumatization in connection with man-made disasters. However, recently some authors have also discussed the fact that patients who suffered from severe organic diseases (such as polio) as children often suddenly fall into dissociative states in certain situations, as they are unconsciously reminded of previous traumas. Recognizing such conditions and assigning them biographically has proven to be indispensable for the therapeutic process of these patients. Therefore, we have argued in some papers that the approach to such

---

[9] References see original publication by Negele et al. (2015).

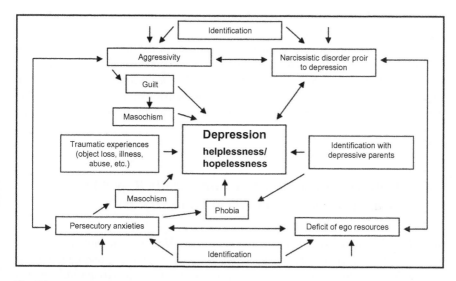

Fig. 7.2 Model of trauma in depression

"historical-biographical truths" (i.e., the reconstruction of traumatizations suffered) is as necessary for the psychological recovery of these patients as the re-experiencing and working through of the traumatizations in the transference relationship with the analyst (cf. in addition, among others, Bohleber & Leuzinger-Bohleber, 2016).

Recognizing and working through traumatization in the treatment process not only is of central importance for those affected but can also help to ensure that the unconscious transmission of traumatization to the next generation can be mitigated and in the best case interrupted, as will be discussed in the following section.

7.7   The Transgenerational Dimension in Psychoanalytic Treatments

Studies from various neighboring disciplines also discuss the connection between trauma and depression and possibilities of transgenerational transmission of family burdens (overview in Böker, 2006). As already discussed in several papers (e.g., in Leuzinger-Bohleber, 2015b), the psychoanalytic knowledge on the short- and long-term effects of severe traumatization comes mainly from clinical work with survivors of the Shoah and their children and grandchildren (cf., e.g., Abraham & Torok 1972/2001; Bose, 1995; Cournut, 1988; Faimberg, 1987; Keilson, 1991; Khan, 1964; Krystal, 1988; Laub, 2005). What the victims of the Shoah experienced exceeds the imagination of all of us. The incomprehensibility of trauma can only be described in a rough approximation in psychoanalytical and scientific terms such as "massive psychic trauma" (cf., e.g., Krystal), sequential (Keilson), or cumulative traumatization (Masud Khan).

Another source of knowledge on the mechanisms of the transgenerational transmission of trauma is studies in the field of epigenetics, which cannot be discussed further in this context (see, e.g., Leuzinger-Bohleber & Fischmann, 2015). Instead, we conclude by illustrating the transgenerative dimension of depression and trauma with two case studies, one from the pilot phase and the other from the main LAC study.

7.8 Identified with a Mother Traumatically Raped by a Soldier in the Second World War (Mrs. B)

Mrs. B. had a depressive breakdown in her early fifties. She was not able to work anymore, was highly suicidal, and suffered from severe sleeping and eating disorders. In her long psychoanalysis, she finally reported that she was sexually abused by her uncle from her 14th to 20th years of life. She had eight abortions during 10 years in her late adolescence often after violent, dangerous sexual experiences which she unconsciously seemed to look for.

Finally, in her psychoanalysis, it was understood that the sexual abuse as well as her dangerous sexual acting out during her late adolescence unconsciously— among others—were connected to embodied memories of a violent rape which she had witnessed as a 3-year-old kid. Her mother was raped in 1945 by Russian soldiers after the occupation of Berlin. The mother was severely traumatized and depressed after this event as well as due to other traumatizations during the Second World War. To mention just one detail: after she got the message that her husband was missed at the Russian front in 1942, she had a psychic breakdown and had to be hospitalized. Her baby, Mrs. B., had to be taken care by her grandmother, a hard and convinced National Socialist who, according to the educational philosophy of that time, refused to emphasize with the basic "weak" needs of her granddaughter. Thus, Mrs. B.—another "child of the war"—also had an early separation trauma. She also was unconsciously identified with her depressed primary object and suffered from heavy guilt feelings and the unconscious conviction that she did not deserve living her own life, having her own children, and being happier than her depressed and traumatized mother.

I have described the complex unconscious determinants of the severe depression of Mrs. B. extensively in another paper (Leuzinger-Bohleber, 2018, p. 134 ff.). In this context, I only want to support the findings of the studies just mentioned that sexual abuse in connection with other early childhood trauma had been central unconscious causes for the severe depression of Mrs. M. even decades later.

7.9   My Parents as well as My Son Were Lying with Me on the Couch ..." (Mr. X)

The transgenerational dimension in the psychoanalysis with Mr. X was particularly impressive. He had been suffering from severe depression for 25 years and belonged to the group of patients who do not seem to be helped by short therapies and most psychotropic drugs and whose relapses of the depression repeat themselves at ever shorter intervals and increase in intensity. Mr. X is his parents' only child. It is known about his early history that he was a "cry baby." The parents were obviously very helpless and went to a pediatrician who advised them not to pay attention to the baby and to let him cry out ... "This strengthens the lungs ...." In the first months of psychoanalysis, he describes his parents as affectionate and caring and turned toward him, but especially in their dealings with their grandson, it turns out more and more that both have a serious empathy disorder: the mother also suffers from migraine and a quite pronounced obsession to clean. The father also complains about a number of psychosomatic symptoms and, like Mr. X, had a "nervous break-down" in a stress situation at work.

Mr. X comes from a in many respects "typical German family of the twentieth century." Both parents experienced the Second World War as adolescents and still remember vividly how they suffered as children under the rigid National Socialist educational ideology. One of his grandfathers had lost an arm in the First World War. He was irascible and often brutally beat the children. Mr. X's mother had to undergo an intestinal operation when the patient was 4 years old. This was the reasons why her son was given for several weeks to a children's recreation home, which was apparently run according to educational principles still in use from the Nazi era. In psychoanalysis, X found out what a traumatic experience the stay in the home had been for him. In psychoanalysis, it becomes clear that through the traumatic separation from his love objects, he had largely lost the basic trust in his inner objects and his self-agency and lived for years in a dissociative state. In many dreams of the initial phase of psychoanalysis, he experiences himself in danger of death, alone and full of panic fear and despair. Here is just one example:

"I see a badly injured man lying by the side of the road – his intestines are hanging out and everything is drenched of blood ... A helicopter appears. It is still unclear as to whether the man is being shot at, or whether he is being helped. Somebody appears and claims that the man has died. I notice that the man is still alive and that he opens his eyes and says: "Why is nobody coming to my aid?" A woman hands him the lid of a cooking pot – which he is meant to place over the wound ... I wake up in a state of panic ..." (Leuzinger-Bohleber, 2015a, p. 2). Despite the dissociative mental states and his social isolation, X was a good student, first completed an apprenticeship and later a course of study. In adolescence, he had a psychosomatic breakdown, which his parents diagnosed as a growth crisis and tried to help him with a vitamin cure. At the age of 15, he found his first girl-friend. His condition improved. But when he separated from her at the age of 22, this triggered—completely unexpected for him—severe psychosomatic reactions.

When his girlfriends separated later, they intensified, until he finally suffered a dramatic breakdown at a party in honor of a new girlfriend: he had to be admitted to the clinic because of hyperventilation (panic attack).

At the beginning of psychoanalysis, he was married to a woman from a non-European country and had a 3½-year-old son. The last severe depression (2½ years ago) was triggered when his wife, in a state of physical exhaustion, attacked him coldly and unempathically after months of double strain due to the renovation of the shared apartment and accused him of endangering his son's life because he crawled toward an open paint can. Mr. X could not defend himself against this attack. The next morning, he awoke with a severe, unbearable depression.

The son is literally lying on the couch. Impressively, it is the patient's relationship to his son that shows his analyst after 3 months that psychoanalysis has an effect on Mr. X. These weeks are characterized by violent acts of aggressive-destructive conflict in his marriage. The little son is often exposed to extremely aggressive conflicts between the parents. The dynamics of the first weeks fill me with great concern and doubt as to whether psychoanalysis can really reach Mr. P.'s inner world. To my astonishment, Mr. X finally managed, after 3 months of treatment, to get the now almost 4-year-old son to sit on the potty and renounce his diaper, a hint for me that Mr. P. can somehow use psychoanalysis to strengthen his fatherly functions. At this time, his son seems to represent a kind of self-object of the patient: in the panic and the desperate cry of the child, Mr. X recognizes his own affects as a child and at the same time seeks the experience that he is able to comfort and calm the little one, a beginning attempt to differentiate between his infantile, traumatized self and the adult one.

When his wife leaves him and his son after 3 months of treatment because of a sexual affair, he is flooded with panic and despair, can hardly sleep, and needs his parents to take care of his son. Surprisingly, the child comes to rest during these weeks and, according to the kindergarten teachers, develops positively: he overcomes his selective mutism and carefully begins to find his way out of his social isolation.

The process of differentiation between self- and object representation seems to develop continuously. Around the middle of the second year of treatment, Mr. X tells the following dream:

> We were on a walk in the forest. A kind of teddy bear accompanied us. Suddenly the bear turned into a dangerous lion. I grabbed the son and fled. The lion followed us. At the last moment I found shelter in a doghouse - I could hardly fit in ...

The associations show that he flees together with his son to the "children's hut" and "leaves the woman to the lion to eat"—a dream image that Mr. X can place in connection with his desire for revenge and death against his wife (but also against his primary objects and me as a transference figure). The dream image again contains the lack of inner separation from his son, who at this time still seems to be predominantly an infantile alter ego, or a narcissistic self-object of the analysand.

In the course of the treatment, inner boundaries between him and his son gradually stabilize. It seems to me that this makes it possible to release the son increasingly from a transgenerational obligation to repeat. Although he—con-sciously—has always protected the son from separations in order not to expect him to suffer a similar separation trauma as he himself experienced it, he could only inadequately develop a trialogue (concept from Dieter Bürgin and Kai von Klitzing) with his baby and his mother and thus support him as an early triangulating object or later during the oedipal phase in the separation from the motherly primary object, which is probably one of the reasons why his son—like the patient—devel-oped into a dreamy, socially withdrawn, anxious latency child.

Decisive for a progressive development is, among other things, the recognition and working through of ambivalent feelings toward his objects—in the third year of treatment, he tells a frightening nightmare in which he sees the body of his son swimming past in an aquarium. The associations lead to his death wishes toward his son. "Without him I would have divorced my wife a long time ago and started a new life—sometimes I feel as dependent on him as I did as a small child on my par-ents who put me in a home …."

Another dream from the third year of psychoanalysis illustrates the inner trans-formations of his relationship to his son:

> *I was in kindergarten. There were many children there - a warm, lively atmosphere. A boy sat on my lap - we joked with each other like men do with each other. I hugged him. To my surprise, it wasn't my son, it was another boy. My son's teacher was also present. He was full of admiration when he watched me - I was very happy. But suddenly I looked more closely at the boy and saw beetles and a black spider crawling out of his eyes - it was ter-rible, scary and threatening, the boy was completely transformed. He looked pale and ill and had deep dark rings under his eyes. - I was shocked and woke up, panic-stricken …*

His first association is as follows: "The eyes are the window to the soul …" Then the abrupt mood swings of his wife occur to him. A few weeks ago, after a long hesi-tation, he finally went to a public educational counselling center, because his son, now almost 10 years old, was still sleeping in his mother's bed. He himself had not been in a position to set boundaries to his wife's overwhelming and seductive behavior. The counsellor described his wife as having a borderline personality, since from one moment to the next, she could transform herself from a charming, gentle woman into a raging, screeching, and violent witch who lost control of her-self and her affects …."

"And in a dream, a relaxed, happy atmosphere suddenly turns into a threatening, horrible, and repulsive situation—the normal, lovable boy mutated into a very sick child. Could it be that you are unconsciously worried that your son might get as sick as your wife?" (Analyst). Mr. X was silent before finally saying: "At the same time, I think that the boy in the dream could also be a part of me … Suddenly I am over-whelmed by my unbearable chronic whole body pain and feel like a miserable, seri-ously ill and helpless child …."

In the following sessions, we carefully approach the previously unbearable inner truth that not only his wife is seriously ill and often loses control over herself and her affects, but that he himself carries within him an analogous, threatening, eerie, and dangerous inner world—which harbors black spiders and hideous insects. Gradually, it becomes possible to recognize and understand the projections and projective identifications in his relationship to his wife—and also to the analyst. Only now is it possible for Mr. X to perceive his own archaic impulses and death wishes toward women, who had often appeared in his dreams, and to integrate them at least partially psychically (cf. Leuzinger-Bohleber, 2015a).

7.10   Some Further Remarks on the Transgenerational Transmission of Trauma

Regular high-frequency psychoanalysis ended after a good 5 years. Since the marriage situation worsens dramatically shortly after the end of the psychoanalysis, we arranged further weekly session (often by phone) which enabled me to receive regular information on the further development of Mr. X and his son.

In brief:

The marital relationship sometimes reminded me of a communicating tube: the more stable Mr. X felt, the more unstable his wife became. She increasingly developed the image of a manifest borderline personality. Again there were frequent scenes of violence: finally, Mrs. X attacked her husband with a knife so that he called the police, and Mrs. X was admitted to the psychiatric clinic. Finally, she accepted medication …. During the following weeks, Mr. X's self-esteem was determined by his ability to cope with "real life with a child." "I'm no longer the little child who collapses completely without his mother and can't get anything together anymore …."

The real separation from his sick mother led to an impressive development of the son. He overcame the secondary enuresis he had been suffering from for a year, a symptom that had strikingly intensified his shyness, social withdrawal, and retreat into an increasingly dangerous computer gaming addiction. This was, in my opinion, related to his mother's difficulty in releasing him from a pathological relationship with her. Mr. X's helplessness in supporting his son in his process of separation from his primary object was probably another reason for the transgenerational transmission of his separation trauma to his son, so now, 6 years after the beginning of his psychoanalysis—Mr. X's observation of his son's progressive development was an important motive for initiating divorce despite serious feelings of guilt and the still massive fears of separation. The wife was admitted to a psychiatric institution and cared for by social workers and psychiatrists. The Youth Welfare Office offered the son play psychotherapy in combination with regular discussions with his parents.

This support facilitated the son's transition to a very ambitious high school (Gymnasium). Despite initial difficulties, especially with his classmates, he was able to master this demanding school and showed increasingly better school performance. This led to a surprisingly good coping with puberty and a visible stabilization of his self-esteem. Together with his father, he regularly visited his mentally ill mother, but he showed a clear outer (and presumably at the same time) inner demar-cation from her.

It was impressive how he transformed his threatening computer game addiction into part of his adolescent identity development: he took part in nationwide compe-titions for a particular computer game, achieved successes, made contact with peers, and developed autonomous abilities (e.g., traveling alone, organizing compe-titions autonomously, etc.).

In the last few months (he is now 15 years old), he has expressed his own vision of his future to his father: he wants to get rich (in contrast to his father, who con-stantly has financial difficulties). A few weeks later, he decides to give up his gam-bling addiction altogether and instead devotes himself to an alternative "scientific project." In order to get rich, but also "to save the world," he had the idea of using hurricanes to generate alternative electricity.

These visions of the future bear the traits of a "normal" adolescent identity-finding process, on the one hand still shaped by fantasies of omnipotence, but on the other hand quite connected with an attempt at integration of specific talents and competences, impulses to differentiate oneself from the primary objects, and one's own visions inspired by the peers. In addition, X was able to use the resurgence of oedipal fantasies and conflicts despite the divorce of his parents and their mental illnesses and vulnerabilities in early adolescence to detach himself from oedipal objects in external reality, but presumably also in internal reality, and to stabilize the boundaries between self- and object representation.

This development of the son relieved Mr. X: "Without the possibility to under-stand and work though my separation trauma in psychoanalysis, I could hardly have let go of my son internally. Moreover, a divorce from my wife would not have been possible ... perhaps my son would then have become as mentally ill as his mother ...," he said.

I agree with Mr. X in my clinical impression. However, this impression can hardly be supported "objectively" or empirically according to the criteria of evidence-based medicine.

7.11 Final Remarks

In a zeitgeist of "faster, more efficient, and cheaper," fantasies of omnipotence are stimulated by health politicians, but also by researchers and therapists, to use effi-cient, "evidence-based" therapeutic techniques to make mental suffering disappear quickly and permanently. Some individuals, e.g., those who suffer from chronic depression due to early severe traumatization, seem to unconsciously oppose this zeitgeist. Thus, various recent studies show that these patients need longer and more intensive treatments in order to be able to live with the enormous mental suffering and not to unconsciously pass it on to their children and grandchildren. As discussed and illustrated in this chapter, intensive psychoanalytic treatments often help to cut the unconscious umbilical cord between the generations. As many of the patients reported both in the DPV outcome study and in the LAC study, one of the most important outcomes of their psychoanalytic therapies was for these patients that they were able to recognize these transgenerative shadows and thus brighten them. "I am infinitely grateful that I no longer have to transmit the misery of our family to our children - and could release them, at least a little bit, from our German war fate of the 20th century ..." (Mrs. S.).

References

Abbass, A., Kisely, S., & Kroenke, K. (2009). Short-term psychodynamic psychotherapy for somatic disorders: Systematic review and meta-analysis of clinical trials. *Psychotherapy and Psychosomatics, 78*, 265–274.

Abraham, N., & Torok, M. (2001). Trauer oder Melancholie. Introjizieren – Inkorporieren. *Psyche-Z Psychoanal, 55*(6), 545–559.

Arnow, B. A., Blasely, C. M., Hunkeler, E. M., Lee, J., & Hayward, C. (2012). Does gender moderate the relationship between childhood maltreatment and adult depression? *Child Maltreatment, 16*, 175–183.

Beutel, M., Leuzinger-Bohleber, M., Rüger, B., Bahrke, U., Negele, A., Haselbacher, A., ... Hautzinger, M. (2012). Psychoanalytic and cognitive-behavior therapy of chronic depression: Study protocol for a randomized controlled trial. *Trials, 13*, 117. Retrieved from http://www.trialsjournal.com/content/pdf/1745-6215-13-117.pdf

Blatt, S. J. (2004). *Experiences of depression: Theoretical, clinical, and research perspectives.* Washington, DC: American Psychological Association.

Blatt, S. J., & Zuroff, D. C. (2005). Empirical evaluation of the assumptions in identifying evidence based treatments in mental health. *Clinical Psychology Review, 25*(4), 459–486.

Bleichmar, H. B. (1996). Some subtypes of depression and their implications for psychoanalytic treatment. *The International Journal of Psycho-Analysis, 77*, 935–961.

Blomberg, J. (2001). Long-term outcome of long-term psychoanalytically oriented therapies: First findings of the Stockholm outcome of psychotherapy and psychoanalysis study. *Psychotherapy Research, 11*(4), 361–382.

Bohleber, W. (2005). Editorial zu the Special Issue oft he Journal Psyche "Depression. Psychoanalytische Erkundungen einer Zeitkrankheit". Zur Psychoanalyse der Depression. Erscheinungsformen-Behandlung-Erklärungsansätze. *Psyche-Z Psychoanal, 59*, 781–788.

Bohleber, W. (2010). *Destructiveness, intersubjectivity, and trauma: the identity crisis of modern psychoanalysis.* London: Karnac.

Bohleber, W., & Leuzinger-Bohleber, M. (2016). The special problem of interpretation in the treatment of traumatized patients. *Psychoanalytic Inquiry, 36*(1), 60–76.

Böker, H. (Ed.). (2006). *Psychoanalyse und Psychiatrie. Geschichte, Krankheitsmodelle und Therapiepraxis.* Heidelberg: Springer.

Bose, J. (1995). Trauma, depression, and mourning. *Contemporary Psychoanalysis, 31*, 399–407.

Bowlby, J. (1980). *Attachment and loss: Vol 3. Loss: Sadness and depression.* New York, NY: Basic Books.

Briere, J. N., & Elliott, D. M. (1994). Immediate and long-term impacts of child sexual abuse. *The Future of Children, 4*, 54–69.

Bromet, E., Andrade, L., Hwang, I., Sampson, N., Alonso, J., de Girolamo, G., ... Kessler, R. (2011). Cross-national epidemiology of DSM-IV major depressive episode. *BMC Medicine, 9*(1), 90. https://doi.org/10.1186/1741-7015-9-90

Corveleyn, J., Luyten, P., Blatt, S. J., & Lens-Gielis, H. (Eds.). (2013). *The theory and treatment of depression: Towards a dynamic interactionism model* (Vol. 5). London: Routledge.

Cournut, J. (1988). Ein Rest, der verbindet. Das unbewußte Schuldgefühl, das Entlehnte betreffend. *Jahrbuch der Psychoanalyse, 22,* 67–99.

Cuipers, P., Huibers, M., & Furukawa, T. (2017). The need for research on treatments of chronic depression. *JAMA Psychiatry, 74,* 242–243.

De Maat, S., de Jonghe, F., de Kraker, R., Leichsenring, F., Abbass, A., Luyten, P., … Dekker, J. (2013). The current state of the empirical evidence for psychoanalysis: A meta-analytic approach. *Harvard Review of Psychiatry, 21,* 107–137.

Driessen, E., Cuijpers, P., de Maat, S., Abbass, A., de Jonghe, F., & Dekker, J. (2010). The efficacy of short-term psychodynamic psychotherapy for depression: A meta-analysis. *Clinical Psychology Review, 30*(1), 25–36.

Ehrenberg, A. (2016). *The weariness of the self: Diagnosing the history of depression in the contemporary age.* Montreal, QC: McGill-Queen's Press-MQUP.

Faimberg, H. (1987). Das Ineinanderrücken der Generationen. Zur Genealogie gewisser Identifizierungen. *Jahrbuch der Psychoanalyse, 20,* 114–143.

Fischer, G., & Riedesser, P. (2009). *Lehrbuch der Psychotraumatologie.* München: Ernst Reinhardt Verlag.

Fonagy, P. (2015). The effectiveness of psychodynamic psychotherapies: An update. *World Psychiatry, 14,* 137–150.

Fonagy, P., Luyten, P., & Allison, E. (2015). Epistemic petrification and the restoration of epistemic trust: A new conceptualization of borderline personality disorder and its psychosocial treatment. *Journal of Personality Disorders, 29*(5), 575–609.

Fonagy, P., Rost, F., Carlyle, J., McPherson, S., Thomas, R., Pasco Fearon, R., … Taylor, D. (2015). Pragmatic randomized controlled trial of long-term psychoanalytic psychotherapy for treatment-resistant depression: The Tavistock Adult Depression Study (TADS). *World Psychiatry, 14*(3), 312–321.

Gibb, B. E., & Alloy, L. B. (2006). A prospective test of the hopelessness theory of depression in children. *Journal of Clinical Child and Adolescent Psychology, 35,* 264–274.

Grande, T., Dilg, R., Jakobsen, T., Keller, W., Krawietz, B., Langer, M., … Rudolf, G. (2009). Structural change as a predictor of long-term follow-up outcome. *Psychotherapy Research, 19*(3), 344–357.

Häuser, W., Schmutzer, G., Brähler, E., & Glaesmer, H. (2011). Misshandlungen in Kindheit und Jugend. Ergebnisse einer Umfrage in einer repräsentativen Stichprobe der deutschen Bevölkerung. *Deutsches Ärzteblatt, 108,* 287–294.

Herman, J. L. (1992). Complex PTSD: A syndrome in survivors of prolonged and repeated trauma. *Journal of Traumatic Stress, 5,* 377–391.

Hill, J. (2009). Developmental perspectives on adult depression. *Psychoanalytic Psychotherapy, 23,* 200–212.

Huber, D., & Klug, G. (2016). Münchner Psychotherapiestudie. *Psychotherapeut, 61*(6), 462–467.

Huhn, M., Tardy, M., Spineli, L. M., Kissling, W., Förstl, H., Pitschel-Walz, G., … Leucht, S. (2014). Efficacy of pharmacotherapy and psychotherapy for adult psychiatric disorders: A systematic overview of meta-analyses. *JAMA Psychiatry, 71,* 706–715.

Hung, C. I., Liu, C. Y., & Yang, C. H. (2019). Persistent depressive disorder has long-term negative impacts on depression, anxiety, and somatic symptoms at 10-year follow-up among patients with major depressive disorder. *Journal of Affective Disorders, 243,* 255–261.

Jimenez, J. P. (2019). *The role of early trauma in depression.* Unpublished paper given at the Joseph Sandler Conference in Buenos Aires, May 2019.

Kächele, H., & Thomä, H. (2000). *Lehrbuch der psychoanalytischen Therapie Band 3 Forschung* [Psychoanalytic practice Vol 3 research]. Ulm: Ulmer Textbank (new edition in preparation).

Kaufhold, H., Bahrke, U., Kallenbach, L., Negele, A., Ernst, M., Keller, W., … Beutel, M. (2019). Wie können nachhaltige Veränderungen in Langzeittherapien untersucht werden?

Symptomatische versus strukturelle Veränderungen in der LAC-Depressionsstudie. *Psyche-Z Psychoanal, 73*, 106–133. https://doi.org/10.21706/ps-73-3-106

Keilson, H. (1991). Sequentielle Traumatisierung bei Kindern. Ergebnisse einer Follow-up-Untersuchung. In *Schicksale der Verfolgten* (pp. 98–109). Berlin: Springer.

Khan, M. (1964). Ego distortion, cumulative trauma, and the role of reconstruction in the analytic situation. *The International Journal of Psycho-Analysis, 45*, 272–279.

Klein, D. N., Shankman, S. A., & Rose, S. (2006). Ten-year prospective follow-up study of the naturalistic course of dysthymic disorder and double depression. *American Journal of Psychiatry, 163*(5), 872–880.

Knekt, P., Lindfors, O., Laaksonen, M. A., Renlund, C., Haaramo, P., Härkänen, T., ... Helsinki Psychotherapy Study Group. (2011). Quasi-experimental study on the effectiveness of psychoanalysis, long-term and short-term psychotherapy on psychiatric symptoms, work ability and functional capacity during a 5-year follow-up. *Journal of Affective Disorders, 13*, 37–47.

Krystal, H. (1988). Integration and self-healing. In *Affect, trauma, alexithymia*. Hillsdale, NJ: The Analytic Press.

Lampe, A. (2002). Die Prävalenz von sexuellem Missbrauch, körperlicher Gewalt und emotionaler Vernachlässigung in der Kindheit in Europa. *Zeitschrift für Psychosomatische Medizin und Psychotherapie, 48*, 370–380.

Lane, R., Ryan, L., Nadel, L., & Greenberg, L. (2015). Memory reconsolidation, emotional arousal, and the process of change in psychotherapy: New insights from brain science. *Behavioral and Brain Sciences, 38*, e1.

Laub, D. (2005). From speechlessness to narrative: The cases of Holocaust historians and of psychiatrically hospitalized survivors. *Literature and Medicine, 24*(2), 253–265.

Leichsenring, F. (2008). Effectiveness of long-term psychodynamic psychotherapy. *Journal of the American Medical Association, 300*(13), 1551–1565.

Leichsenring, F., & Rabung, S. (2011). Long-term psychodynamic psychotherapy in complex mental disorders: Update of a meta-analysis. *British Journal of Psychiatry, 199*, 15–22.

Leuzinger-Bohleber, M. (2005). Chronifizierende Depression: Eine Indikation für Psychoanalysen und psychoanalytische Langzeittherapien. *Psyche-Z Psychoanal, 59*, 789–815.

Leuzinger-Bohleber, M. (2015a). *Finding the body in the mind – Embodied memories, trauma, and depression*. International Psychoanalytical Association. London: Karnac.

Leuzinger-Bohleber, M. (2015b). Working with severely traumatized, chronically depressed analysands. *International Journal of Psycho-Analysis, 96*, 611–636.

Leuzinger-Bohleber, M., Arnold, S., & Kaechele, H. (Eds.). (2015/2019). *An open door review of outcome and process studies in psychoanalysis*. London: International Psychoanalytical Association. Retrieved from https://www.ipa.world/

Leuzinger-Bohleber, M., & Fischmann, T. (2015). Transgenerationelle Weitergabe von Trauma und Depression: Psychoanalytische und epigenetische Überlegungen. In V. Lux & J. T. Richter (Eds.), *Kulturen der Epigenetik: Vererbt, Codiert, Übertragen* (pp. 69–88). Berlin: De Gruyter.

Leuzinger-Bohleber, M., Hautzinger, M., Fiedler, G., Keller, W., Bahrke, U., Kallenbach, L., ... Küchenhoff, H. (2019). Outcome of psychoanalytic and cognitive-behavioural long-term therapy with chronically depressed patients: A controlled trial with preferential and randomized allocation. *The Canadian Journal of Psychiatry, 64*(1), 47–58.

Leuzinger-Bohleber, M., Kallenbach, L., Bahrke, U., Kaufhold, J., Negele, A., Ernst, M., ... Beutel, M. E. (2020). The LAC study: A comparative outcome study of psychoanalytic and cognitive-behavioral long-term, therapies of chronic depressive patients. In M. Leuzinger-Bohleber, M. Solms, & S. E. Arnold (Eds.), *Outcome research and the future of psychoanalysis. Clinicans and researchers in dialogue* (pp. 136–166). London: Routledge.

Leuzinger-Bohleber, M., Kaufhold, J., Kallenbach, L., Negele, A., Ernst, M., Keller, W., ... Beutel, M. (2019). How to measure sustained psychic transformations in long-term treatments of chronically depressed patients: Symptomatic and structural changes in the LAC Depression Study of the outcome of cognitive-behavioural and psychoanalytic long-term treatments. *International Journal of Psycho-Analysis, 100*(1), 99–127.

Leuzinger-Bohleber, M., Solms, M., & Arnold, S. E. (Eds.). (2020). *Outcome research and the future of psychoanalysis. Clinicians and researchers in dialogue*. London: Routledge.

Leuzinger-Bohleber, M., Stuhr, U., Rüger, B., & Beutel, M. (2003). How to study the 'quality of psychoanalytic treatments' and their long-term effects on patients' well-being: A representative, multi-perspective follow-up study. *International Journal of Psycho-Analysis, 84*(2), 263–290.

Liliengren, P. (2019). *Comprehensive compilation of randomized controlled trials, RCTs, involving psychodynamic treatment and interventions*. Retrieved from https://www.research-gate.net/pulication/317335876

McGrath, E., Keita, G. P., Stickland, B. R., & Russo, N. F. (1993). *Frauen und Depression: Risikofaktoren und Behandlungsfragen*. Bergheim: Meckinger Verlag.

Molnar, B. E., Buka, S. L., & Kessler, R. C. (2001). Child sexual abuse and subsequent psychopathology: Results from the national comorbidity survey. *American Journal of Public Health, 91*, 753–760.

Murphy, J. A., & Byrne, G. J. (2012). Prevalence and correlates of the proposed DSM-5 diagnosis of chronic depressive disorder. *Journal of Affective Disorders, 139*(2), 172–180.

Negele, A., Kaufhold, J., Kallenbach, L., & Leuzinger-Bohleber, M. (2015). Childhood trauma and its relation to chronic depression in adulthood. *Depression Research and Treatment, 2015*, 650804.

Peterson, B., Leuzinger-Bohleber, M., Fischmann, T, Ambresin, G., Axmacher, N., & Lerner, R. et al. (2019). *Multi-level outcome study of psychoanalyses of chronically depressed patients with early trauma (MODE) -- Initial phase*. Unpublished Research Application to the IPA/ApsaA.

Rudolf, G., Jakobsen, T., Keller, W., Krawietz, B., Langer, M., Oberbracht, C., ... Grande, T. (2012). Umstrukturierung als Ergebnisparadigma der psychodynamischen Psychotherapie - Ergebnisse aus der Praxisstudie Analytische Langzeittherapie. *Zeitschrift für Psychosomatische Medizin und Psychotherapie, 58*(1), 55–66.

Scher, D., Forde, D. R., McQuaid, J. R., & Stein, M. B. (2004). Prevalence and demographic correlates of childhood maltreatment in an adult community sample. *Child Abuse & Neglect, 28*, 167–180.

Shedler, J. (2010). The efficacy of psychodynamic psychotherapy. *American Psychologist, 65*, 98–109.

Shedler, J. (2015). Where is the evidence for "evidence-based" therapy? *The Journal of Psychological Therapies in Primary Care., 4*, 47–59.

Spijker, J., van Straten, A., Bockting, C. L., Meeuwissen, J. A., & van Balkom, A. J. (2013). Psychotherapy, anti-depressants, and their combination for chronic major depressive disorder: A systematic review. *Canadian Journal of Psychiatry, 58*, 386–392.

Steinert, C., Hofmann, M., Kruse, J., & Leichsenring, F. (2014). Relapse rates after psychotherapy for depression - Stable long-term effects? A meta-analysis. *Journal of Affective Disorders, 168*, 107–18.2002.

Taylor, D. (2010). Tavistock-Manual der Psychoanalytischen Psychotherapie. *Psyche-Z Psychoanal, 64*, 833–886.

Teicher, M. H., Samson, J. A., Polcari, A., & Andersen, S. L. (2009). Length of time between onset of childhood sexual abuse and emergence of depression in a young adult sample: A retrospective clinical report. *Journal of Clinical Psychiatry, 70*, 684–691.

Trivedi, R. B., Nieuwsma, J. A., & Williams, J. W. (2011). Examination of the utility of psychotherapy for patients with treatment resistant depression: A systematic review. *Journal of General Internal Medicine, 26*, 643–650.

van der Kolk, B. (2005). Developmental trauma disorder. *Psychiatric Annals, 35*, 401–408.

Vandeleur, C. L., Fassassi, S., Castelao, E., Glaus, J., Strippoli, M. P. F., Lasserre, A. M., ... Angst, J. (2017). Prevalence and correlates of DSM-5 major depressive and related disorders in the community. *Psychiatry Research, 250*, 50–58.

Wetzel, P. (1998). Gewalterfahrungen in der Kindheit. In *Sexueller Missbrauch, körperliche Misshandlung und deren langfristige Konsequenzen*. Baden-Baden: Nomos.

Widom, C. S., DuMont, K., & Czaja, S. (2007). A prospective investigation of major depressive disorder and comorbidity in abused and neglected children grown up. *Archives of General Psychiatry, 64*, 49–56.

World Health Organization. (2013/2017). *The global burden of disease: 2004 Update*. Geneva: Author. Retrieved from http://www.who.int/healthinfo/global_burden_disease/GBD_report_2004update_full.pdf

Chapter 8
Major Depression: A Cognitive-Behavioral Perspective to Pathology, Case Conceptualization, and Treatment

Georgia Panayiotou

Contents

Major depressive disorder is a common, often chronic, and debilitating condition affecting millions of individuals of all ages around the globe. The suffering experienced by about 7% of the population in the USA and Europe and over 264 million people of all ages worldwide (WHO, 2020) contributes to the economic and societal burden incurred by mental disorders, due to loss of productivity, unemployment, and healthcare seeking. Although the majority of patients suffering from depression do not attempt or commit suicide, this particular disorder is one of the most significant proximal predictors of suicide risk. For all these reasons, and for the tremendous impact of major depression on the quality of life and health of individuals, families, and societies (Wittchen et al., 2011), its etiology and treatment has been the focus of attention for many researchers. They have contributed significant evidence regarding its biological, social, and psychological predictors and the effectiveness of various modes of pharmacological and behavioral therapies. This chapter summarizes some of the current evidence regarding the etiological and maintenance factors in major depression, with an emphasis on the psychological perspective associated with cognitive-behavioral therapy (CBT), and delineates the major treatment components of this approach.

Major depressive disorder, as described in the DSM-5, has an episodic course, characterized by periodic major depressive episodes, that, when untreated, can last

G. Panayiotou (✉)

Department of Psychology and Center of Applied Neuroscience, University of Cyprus, Nicosia, Cyprus

e-mail: georgiap@upcy.ap.cy

© Springer Nature Switzerland AG 2021   107
C. Charis, G. Panayiotou (eds.), *Depression Conceptualization and Treatment*,
https://doi.org/10.1007/978-3-030-68932-2_8

for several months to over a year (Whiteford et al., 2013) with estimates varying in different studies, interrupted by periods of full or partial remission. Major depressive disorder or unipolar depression, as it is also referred to, consists of only depressive episodes without manic or hypomanic episodes, the presence of which warrants a different diagnosis. Specifically, a major depressive episode can be diagnosed if five (or more) of the following symptoms are present during a 2-week period, representing a change from typical functioning (APA, 2013): The primary symptoms are either (1) depressed mood or (2) loss of interest or pleasure, where either one or two occur for most of the day, nearly every day. These primary symptoms must be accompanied by at least four of the following: (3) significant weight loss or weight gain or significant changes in appetite, (4) insomnia or hypersomnia, (5) slowing down of thought and reduced physical movement, (6) fatigue or loss of energy, (7) feelings of worthlessness or excessive guilt, (8) diminished ability to think or concentrate or indecisiveness, and (9) recurrent thoughts of death, suicidal ideation, or a suicide attempt or plan. Notably, for children and adolescents, the predominant mood can be irritable rather than depressed, and weight changes can be substituted by absence of appropriate weight gain. As in the case of other DSM-5 disorders, these symptoms cannot be better explained by a medical condition, or a different disorder, are not the outcome of medications or substances, and cause significant impairment in functioning. DSM-5 also lists a number of specifiers and subtypes, as no two individuals with depression appear to have exactly the same clinical presentation.

A milder and more chronic form of depression, dysthymia, is diagnosed when the depressed mood or loss of interest lasts for at least 2 years in adults (one in children and adolescents) and includes at least two symptoms similar to those described for major depression (i.e., changes in eating/appetite, sleep, low energy or fatigue, low self-esteem, concentration or decision-making difficulty, hopelessness).

Major depression has its onset predominantly in the early adult years (APA, 2013), but adolescents (Costello, Erkanli, & Angold, 2006) and the elderly (Palsson & Skoog, 1997) are also at heightened risk. Notably, as will be discussed later, this is a mainly female disorder, with women being 1.5–3 times more likely to suffer from it, with gender differences already apparent by adolescence (APA, 2013).

8.1 The Psychopathology of Depression

The cognitive-behavioral perspective understands depression as stemming from the interaction of dispositional vulnerabilities, i.e., heredity and temperament, with cognitive characteristics (learned, or inherited) that have to do with how the world is understood and processed. Recent advances in genetic research have shown that major depression risk is to a significant degree heritable, with a heritability rate for about 37%. Although many genes have been shown to have associations with depression, there is no clear picture at this point of a specific genetic substrate for this disorder (or for most other psychiatric disorders). For example, a recent, large genome-wide association study on major depressive disorder identified numerous genetic variants associated with depression (Wray et al., 2018), but none unique and specific to it. In part, this may be due to the large heterogeneity within the population of depressed individuals, both in symptoms and in developmental trajectories of depression (Dekker et al., 2007).

To address the heterogeneity observed among those suffering from this disorder, research has also focused on identifying behavioral endophenotypes for depression (Gottesman & Gould, 2003), i.e., heritable characteristics that form part of the mechanism linking genes to disease expression. Promising endophenotypes, found more strongly in families of patients with depression compared to the general population, include neuroticism, decreased sensitivity of the reward system, harm avoidance, decreased cognitive control, negative affectivity, and behavioral inhibition. Research on such predisposing temperament and personality factors remains inconclusive, however, given measurement issues, and the relative dearth of longitudinal research (Lim, Barlas, & Ho, 2018) and twin studies. Some evidence suggests only modest to moderate genetic association between major depression, neuroticism, and self-reported depressive symptoms (Kendler, Gatz, Gardner, & Pedersen, 2006; Kendler & Myers, 2010), with the latter potentially representing a different factor more closely related to either transient negative affect or a milder, chronic depressive style (Kendler et al., 2019), rather than with true, episodic expressions of major depression.

A core characteristic that seems to be the most proximal predictor of depression is a negative thinking style (Alloy et al., 2000; Panayiotou & Papageorgiou, 2007) that includes a propensity toward rumination, negative attributions and interpretations, self-focused attention on negative aspects of the self, self-blame, and increased over-general memory especially of negative personal events. According to the cognitive vulnerability hypothesis (e.g., Alloy, Abramson, Walshaw, & Neeren, 2006), people who are vulnerable to either depressive symptoms or major depressive episodes have a specific, negative attribution style. They interpret negative events as caused by themselves, and by stable and global factors (including their own flawed characteristics). This negative thought content is caused or at least maintained by a series of well-established cognitive biases in the way information is processed by depressed individuals, both adults and children/adolescents. Cognitive biases underlie the preferential processing of negative information in various disorders; however, in addition to this negativity bias, there also seems to be an absence of the more normative positivity bias in depressed people (Armstrong & Olatunji, 2012; Peckham, McHugh, & Otto, 2010). The fact that these biases exist, according to some evidence, in non-symptomatic children of depressed parents (Kujawa et al., 2011), and among individuals without depression who later develop symptoms, suggests that they play a causative role in the pathogenesis of depression (Everaert, Koster, & Derakshan, 2012). However, more research is needed to establish these as true endophenotypes, as heritability studies are limited (Goldstein & Klein, 2014). These biases, whether acquired or inherited, include, more specifically, the preferential attention to negative information, negative interpretations of ambiguous information (Wisco & Nolen-Hoeksema, 2010), and enhanced memory for negative content (Koster, De Raedt, Leyman, & De Lissnyder, 2010; Peckham et al., 2010). Their persistence may be sustained by poor executive control that leads to failure of disengagement and inhibition of depressive thought content (Joormann, Yoon, & Zetsche, 2007).

With regard to attention biases, these appear to involve primarily difficulty in disengagement from negative information, rather than increased selective attention to negative stimuli (De Raedt & Koster, 2010), with the latter being more common in anxiety. Correspondingly, the pattern of attentional avoidance of negative information often seen in anxious individuals is not typically observed in depression. Interpretation biases pertain especially to ambiguous self-relevant information (Wisco & Nolen-Hoeksema, 2010), which is interpreted in a negative, self-deprecating light. Concerning memory biases, depressed individuals tend to recall over-general and negative memories compared to non-depressed individuals (e.g., Williams et al., 2007). These ways of processing information about the world, the self, and the future seem to interact and feed into each other (Everaert et al., 2012), playing a crucial role in maintaining negative content in awareness and making the world appear hopeless and threatening. Although CBT treatments initially focused more on the content of thought, rather than on the way information is processed, such empirical evidence from basic science is progressively informing CBT, leading to experimentation with promising therapeutic components like attention bias modification (e.g., Beevers, Clasen, Enock, & Schnyer, 2015; Yang, Ding, Dai, Peng, & Zhang, 2015) and cognitive bias modification therapy (e.g., Joormann, Waugh, & Gotlib, 2015), either as stand-alone treatments or components of a broader CBT protocol.

It is generally believed that depression episodes in a person with these hereditary, cognitive, and emotional risk characteristics are triggered by stressful life events (Ingram, Miranda, & Segal, 1998), often associated with some type of loss (loved ones, health, way of life, self-esteem) and exposure to such events predicts increased risk for depression, especially among those who experienced early childhood trauma and/or have temperamental risk factors like neuroticism (Kendler, Kuhn, & Prescott, 2004). Depressed individuals report more negative life events than non-depressed people, potentially, in part due to their negatively biased memory and in part because they have actually experienced such events, which may have increased their vulnerability.

In terms of emotional reactivity, depression has been associated with a pattern of hypo-reactive autonomic responses to negative emotional stimulation and sometimes during rest, potentially reflecting apathy, behavioral inactivation, and passive avoidance (Schiweck, Piette, Berckmans, Claes, & Vrieze, 2019). Depression has also been associated with decreased heart rate variability (Carney et al., 2001) suggesting reduced cardiovagal activity (Agelink, Boz, Ullrich, & Andrich, 2002) and poor autonomic flexibility and emotion regulation ability (Panayiotou, Panteli, & Vlemincx, 2019, Panayiotou, 2018). Low skin conductance (Williams, Iacono, & Remick, 1985) has also been associated with depression. Reduced emotional reactivity may be indicative of a learned helplessness pattern of responses and physiological and behavioral immobilization (Porges, 2001), where one has learned that no action will result in positive outcomes (Panayiotou, 2018).

An important aspect of the psychopathology of depression that may have implications for its etiology and maintenance pertains to the gender disparities in prevalence that characterize this disorder. In childhood, prevalence rates are about equal, or, according to some estimates, boys are more likely to be depressed (Nolen-Hoeksema, 1987). At puberty, there is a dramatic reversal of the statistics, with women being about 50% more likely to develop depression. Many explanations have been given to these disparities, though more research seems to be needed in order to reach definitive conclusions. Biological or genetic factors have not received much research support (Piccinelli & Wilkinson, 2000). Lower power status in society (Bebbington, 1998; Radloff, 1975), unfavorable for women sex roles, socioeconomic status (i.e., greater poverty among women), and social stereotypes, for example, about gender-appropriate ways of coping, have been implicated (Panayiotou & Papageorgiou, 2007). Other environmental factors have been implicated, like the higher prevalence of childhood abuse among women (Brown, 2002) and the fact that women face a multitude of practical difficulties and negative life events, stemming from their multiple social roles (Nolen-Hoeksema, 1991), which include child-rearing and caring for elderly parents. Although the evidence for many of these predictors remains mixed, these contextual vulnerability factors are believed to interact with more proximal characteristics, such as low self-esteem and personality traits, like neuroticism or behavioral inhibition to increase chances of depression in women. It is likely that these environmental risk factors, some of which exist from an early age, play a critical role in shaping stereotypes, attribution style, negative thinking content, and self-defeating behaviors, which according to the cognitive-behavioral model are the central driving force that drives depression for all individuals, including women (Hankin & Abramson, 2001).

A critical cognitive characteristic that may in part explain the gender differences in depression prevalence, and plays a central role in cognitive models of depression (and related disorders, like social anxiety; Panayiotou & Vrana, 1998), is self-focused attention. It appears that ruminative self-focus and self-consciousness (Panayiotou & Kokkinos, 2006), that is, a tendency to focus on and regurgitate negative thoughts and evaluations about the self, is part of a vicious cycle that maintains depression and other emotional disorders. High levels of self-focused attention increase negative affect by directing attention to it, while higher negative affect has been found to increase self-focused attention, by making the self more salient (Panayiotou, Brown, & Vrana, 2007). According to Nolen-Hoeksema (1987) and Nolen, Wisco, and Lyubomirsky (2008), ruminative self-focus increases dysphoric mood and is maintained by negative reinforcement. It provides the depressed person the illusion that one is doing something active: By rethinking the past to identify faults and limitations, the depressed person believes that they are helping their situation, when in fact one does nothing to change one's life and assume responsibility. In essence, self-focused attention is used as an avoidant emotion regulation strategy, known to contribute to many forms of psychopathology (Panayiotou, Karekla, & Leonidou, 2017). Ruminative self-focus is higher in women than men, perhaps because men are socialized to use more active problem-solving, while women may be socialized into more passive roles, talking about their problems and seeking emotional help from others (Panayiotou, Karekla, & Mete, 2014). Such differences in coping may contribute to prevalence differences between genders.

8.2 Cognitive-Behavioral Conceptualization of Depression Etiology and Maintenance

Although cognitive and behavioral theoretical frameworks to the conceptualization and treatment of depression are somewhat distinct, in practice CBT clinicians typically apply protocols incorporating aspects of both perspectives. With each theory emphasizing somewhat different etiological routes to the development and maintenance of depression, ultimately, thoughts, affective reactions, and behaviors and the way they mutually affect each other are central to the understanding and treatment of depression and other affective disorders, as the review above indicates. CBT therapists understand that most individuals seek therapy because of emotional distress. However, as they explain to their clients from the very early sessions of treatment, emotions occur automatically and are difficult to change directly. Because emotions are mutually connected to and mutually influence thoughts and behaviors, change in negative affect and depression is expected to come about after the client is able to modulate and change one's thoughts/interpretations and/or one's behavior. Central to both the cognitive and behavioral perspective is a functional analysis of the client's behavior (including the client's thoughts). Understanding the ABCs that maintain depression, i.e., the Antecedents, Behaviors, and Consequences in repeated chains of depressive behaviors (such as oversleeping, overeating, avoiding social interactions, thinking thoughts like "I'm useless," etc.), provides a window into the individualized maintenance mechanisms of depression. It also provides hypotheses that therapist and client jointly test and experiment with in order to incur therapeutic change. The case formulation (Eells, 2007), in addition to the problem list, precipitants of current problems, and maintenance mechanisms, typically includes identified predisposing factors, both individual and contextual, and the strengths and weaknesses the client brings to therapy that might impact its success (e.g., good vs. poor insight, a supportive vs. unsupportive home environment). Therapy takes place in a collaborative, hypothesis testing, solution-focused approach where therapist and client are active agents of change. As in all therapy, a strong therapeutic alliance and commitment to a shared conceptualization are prerequisites for positive outcomes.

8.2.1 The Behavioral Perspective

The role of behavioral withdrawal, which leads to decreased opportunities for positive reinforcement, plays a central role in the behavioral point of view. This perspective postulates that depressive behaviors, like staying in bed, overeating, ruminating, using substances, and other depressive patterns, are reinforced positively or negatively and maintained by their consequences, which must therefore be closely monitored and identified, a major goal of therapy. Identifying strategies for reducing the reinforcement of depressive behaviors can be an important treatment component (Hopko, Lejuez, Lepage, Hopko, & McNeil, 2003). A fundamental goal of therapy is to modify behavior directly (Dimidjian, Martell, Addis, & Herman-Dunn, 2008) so as to increase the likelihood of positive reinforcement and solve the problems that lead to stress. Although focusing on patterns of behavior and their contingencies in the present, this approach does not ignore the client's history. It suggests that patterns of behavior that prohibit one from living a fulfilling life in the present may have been reinforced and shaped by one's past (traumatic) experiences. Behaviors that should lead to positive consequences may have been extinguished through punishment or non-reinforcement (e.g., Ferster, 1981). This elicits depressed mood, which in turn makes it less likely for the person to emit such behaviors, in order to feel better or solve life problems. Instead, depressed individuals typically engage in self-focused attention and rumination (Nolen-Hoeksema, 1987; Panayiotou & Papageorgiou, 2007) and try to avoid and escape situations that might result in what they predict will be adverse consequences and emotions but may be necessary to enjoy a fulfilling life. Avoidance and withdrawal (of many forms) are conceptualized as coping behaviors, reinforced by the short-term relief they produce; in the long term, however, they keep one away from engaging with important aspects of their lives and relationships. Behavioral activation, the therapeutic approach stemming from this conceptualization, even though more clearly behavioral than cognitive, is a core component in many forms of CBT, including the classical cognitive therapy model for depression as proposed by Beck (1979).

Behavioral activation, as part of a more comprehensive CBT protocol or as a stand-alone brief treatment (Lejuez, Hopko, & Hopko, 2001), has received empirical support for its efficacy (Dimidjian et al., 2006), which was deemed equivalent to antidepressant pharmacotherapy but with longer-lasting effects. By increasing behaviors that may lead to rewards and actively solve life problems, while decreasing avoidance and withdrawal, it aims not to necessarily increase happiness directly and immediately, but to improve wellbeing and quality of life through increased engagement with ones' valued life goals and progressive engagement with rewarding behaviors. This changed context may in turn work to improve mood. Furthermore, the aim of behavioral activation is not, as often misunderstood, to just increase the amount of behavior in general (i.e., go to the gym, sort out one's house). Instead, in a collaborative, systematic, and guided manner, it aims to identify important target behaviors that are valued by the client and facilitate engagement with them. It does so by breaking the behavior down into smaller chunks, or by creating a hierarchy based on the difficulty of execution (Hopko et al., 2003). Client and therapist then identify and resolve obstacles to execution, practice in and outside of session, and increase the probability of success, for example, using prompts and reminders while at the same time acknowledging that the required change is challenging and difficult for the client to implement (Dimidjian et al., 2008). Cognitive rehearsal, i.e., practicing the assignment in one's imagery, may be used to predict difficulties and prepare successful homework completion. In its application the treatment is highly idiographic, in that it is based on the detailed functional analysis of each client's behavioral patterns. Toward this aim, rating scales and record forms are frequently used where the client keeps careful track of their behaviors, often several times a day. Of importance is that the client comprehends and agrees to the rationale for this treatment and engages in it. It is very important that doubts are addressed and the pain of the client is heard. Change is not easy (otherwise the client would have found solutions without therapy), and one should not be made to feel that their distress or vulnerability is not valid. Therapists often find that clients are convinced that they must first feel better and then engage in meaningful behaviors, rather than the other way around. They may in essence be afraid that by being effective in their lives their pain won't be heard—these issues must be addressed with compassion and empathy, and the link between decreased goal-directed behavior and lack of positive outcomes must be clearly understood.

Behavioral activation is based on collaborative exploration of the observations the client makes of their own lives and requires practice and application of what was learned in therapy through between session homework assignments. As in all CBT treatments, homework is very important, empowering the client and making them responsible for their own progress. As such, it is typically reviewed first and extensively as part of the agreed agenda of each session. If goals are not accomplished, careful assessment of the contingencies and circumstances is the focus of the next session to identify obstacles. It is important that unaccomplished goals are not presented as client failure, but rather as due to a goal that was not broken down enough, to obstacles that were not identified, or to prompts and reminders that were not set. It is very important to reformulate and change the assignments, to increase the probability that success will happen. As Beck has put it, the first step in the goal of preparing a meal may involve boiling an egg (Beck, 1979); success is expected to motivate further change. Homework successes are actively praised by the therapist (token economy protocols can be used in inpatient settings; Lejuez et al., 2001), and the patient and therapist fully review the processes that facilitated success. Then the client is called to maintain and/or generalize these new behaviors to ensure that they begin to become part of their behavioral repertoires.

8.2.2   The Cognitive Perspective

From a cognitive perspective as described by the influential work of Ellis (e.g., Ellis, 1957), Beck (e.g., Beck, 1995), Padesky (e.g., Padesky & Greenberger, 2012; Hawley et al., 2017), and others, the interpretation and meaning given to various stressors and events by the individual is typically what instigates negative emotions, and behaviors, which in turn help to perpetuate and reinforce depressogenic cognitions. However, cognitions, emotions, and behaviors mutually affect each other, and therapy must take all three components into account. According to Beck's model, depression involves negative schemas, i.e., mental representations about the self, the world, and the future, called the cognitive triad. These "core beliefs" are activated by stressful life events and lead to "cognitive distortions" or "automatic thoughts" (e.g., regularly catastrophizing, overgeneralizing, etc.) which tend to be repeated across situations. Core beliefs about the self (e.g., perfectionism) hold a central role in depression (Hawley, Ho, Zuroff, & Blatt, 2006), and their modification may be necessary to achieve change, especially for chronic or recurrent symptoms. These central stereotypes are associated with the negatively biased information processing discussed above and form a framework into which the world fits: Information congruent with these schemas is attended to preferentially, the world is interpreted through their filter, and memory is increased for congruent rather than incongruent information. The more these schemas are practiced, by repeated activation in memory, the more they become reinforced and ingrained (Ingram, 1984).

The goal of the cognitive component of CBT is to increase awareness of the role of cognitions and interpretations on mood and behavior, to train the client to identify cognitive distortions, and to come about with more realistic interpretations of situations. The aim is *not* to attach silver linings to difficult situations, but to realize and mitigate the exaggeration, persistent self-blame, and stable, over-general interpretations that often sustain negative thinking. As in all CBT, sessions are relatively structured, following a mutually agreed agenda. Homework is always assigned and discussed. However, room is allowed for patients who may feel the need to briefly discuss something that seems outside the set agenda in order to sustain rapport and show empathy.

Several important tools are used in the process of identifying and challenging dysfunctional cognitions and core beliefs. The Socratic dialogue involves the process of questioning by the therapist about particular depressive situations and cognitions that the client brings into therapy. The goal of elaborate questioning is to direct the client's attention to important details (in light of over-general memory) and to help them discover patterns of thinking and behavior that maintain depression. This process, in addition to focusing questions, involves empathic reflection by the therapist, summary statements, and synthesizing questions that help the client produce their own conclusions about maintenance mechanisms and patterns in their behavior, in a process of "guided discovery" (Kazantzis, Fairburn, Padesky, Reinecke, & Teesson, 2014). Through Socratic dialogue the "downward spiral" (Beck, 1995) of client's negative thinking can be identified. With questions like "What makes this important?", "Why would that matter?", "What would it mean to you if …?", the central fears and concerns of clients can be derived from their generalized statements and ruminations.

Automatic thought records are another crucial tool in CBT. Although various versions of these exist, they are essentially a diary of situations that triggered negative thoughts and emotions and at a later step include the assignment of challenging the thoughts and reappraising the situation. The columns of the record typically include a brief note of the situation, the thoughts that immediately preceded one's emotional reaction, the emotions experienced and their intensity, and finally the rebuttal of the thought with a more balanced, rational one that is produced after the available evidence is weighted. A final column showing the outcome (new interpretation and new emotions) may be included. Much practice in session, modeling by the therapists, and guided discovery by the client is required to effectively identify and correct dysfunctional automatic thoughts. Role-playing, questioning, and imagery can help elicit them. Practice in identifying and weighing the evidence for and against the dysfunctional interpretation, to reach the necessary reappraisal, is encouraged by the therapist. Padesky and Greenberger (2012) suggest that the client must be fully convinced that the evidence is in favor of the new restructured thought and against the distorted one, or the automatic thought will persist. To achieve this conviction, specific columns can be added to the thought record, where evidence for and against an automatic thought are carefully recorded, with persistent exploration of "any other evidence" that still might linger in support of the distortion. Finding out collaboratively with the client, through Socratic questioning and self-discovery, that the evidence does not support the faulty assumption will facilitate change. In all cases, automatic thoughts are treated as hypotheses to be tested. If prior experience is not adequate to provide evidence for or against them, therapist and client design behavioral experiments (i.e., behavioral assignments that directly speak to the assumptions of the automatic thought—e.g., that one will faint if one tries to ask a question in class) to assemble new evidence.

Changing core beliefs, the deeply held stereotypes that permeate many life domains and which were probably reinforced throughout development, is a greater challenge for the CBT therapist and may only need to be undertaken for pervasive and chronic emotional problems, during the final stages of treatment. Core beliefs are difficult to change because they have been created over a lifetime of reinforcement, potentially in the absence of any alternative evidence, and from there on have also shaped the way the world is perceived, understood, and remembered, producing further supportive evidence for their veridicality. Such schemas can be changed using a variety of interventions that aim not only to refute them, but to create new, alternative beliefs to replace them. Various interventions can aid in challenging core beliefs as described in Padesky (1994). The continuum technique involves drawing and discussing continuous dimensions for constructs that are absolute and categorical in the mind of the client, to reinforce flexibility. An example is the use of a "pie chart of blame," where a client who tends to assume that "it was all my fault" is asked to draw a pie chart on which to think of any potential sources of responsibility for a particular problem and add a representative percentage of "blame" on the pie. Through brainstorming of all potential sources of responsibility, a pie is continuously filled in, and the client contemplates about a more realistic portion of the blame that can be attributed to themselves. The positive log technique involves learning to keep note of all evidence that supports a new, more functional schema. Using the historical test for schema technique, the therapist helps the client identify supportive and disconfirming evidence for long-held schemas from the client's own developmental history. Overall, the aim in addressing long-standing core beliefs is to ensure that new evidence against them, which supports alternative and more accurate ideas, is actually believable to the client, who is now asked to radically change their view of the self, the world, and the future.

8.3 Future Directions in CBT and Empirically Validated Treatments

Because of the centrality of cognitive biases in the maintenance of depression, as noted above, specific interventions designed to modify these biases are continuously tested, either as stand-alone treatments or as components of CBT protocols. For example, attention bias modification therapy (ABMT) aims to decrease the probability that an individual will look at and focus attention on negative stimuli while increasing the probability that they will focus on affectively neutral stimuli (or in some cases positive stimuli). This is accomplished through computerized programs that guide the participant to "choose" to look more at neutral stimuli, when these are presented in neutral-negative pairs on the computer screen. ABMT has shown promise for various emotional disorders, including depression (Beevers et al., 2015; Yang et al., 2015), but contradictory evidence also exists, with the literature starting to focus on the moderators that determine its effectiveness (Neophytou, 2019). Cognitive bias modification (CBM) techniques, through computerized tasks, have also been used to change negative interpretation biases, which seem central in maintaining depression (MacLeod & Mathews, 2012; Williams et al., 2015). Although several studies have been implemented with promising results, meta-analyses of existing CBM treatments for adult depression show, at present, small effect sizes (Cristea, Kok, & Cuijpers, 2015). It remains to be seen whether further improvement of these interventions, identification of moderators of effectiveness, or combination with other potent components of CBT will improve overall treatment efficacy.

Other developments pertain to the recent accumulation of neuroscientific evidence, aiming to identify biomarkers of specific dysfunctions in depression and the causes of heterogeneity among those suffering from depressive disorders. With the goal of personalized medicine in mind, it becomes progressively important to precisely identify such deficits and target interventions to the unique causes that may underlie depression in each individual. This could become feasible, through neuroimaging to identify sub-categories of depression patterns, for example, those whose depression stems from a dysfunction of the reward system, with primary symptoms of anhedonia, vs. those whose depression derives from resting-state dysfunction, leading to increased rumination (Williams, 2016).

Other contemporary interventions, rather than focusing on specificity, are more generalized and focus on trans-diagnostic symptoms that are maintained by the same core vulnerabilities mechanisms that are shared, for example, between anxiety, depression, and other emotional disorders (Sauer-Zavala et al., 2017). Similar trans-diagnostic approaches can be taken to address shared risk factors, like emotion dysregulation, that are common across disorders. Providing interventions that train core skills of how to accept, reframe, or problem solve difficult emotional situations appears to hold promise, especially as an early prevention application for those who are at risk for a variety of disorders, including depression (Theodorou, 2020, unpublished dissertation). When discussing contemporary developments, one should also note the multitude of computer-delivered treatments for depression and other disorders that progressively enter the market, often showing equitable effectiveness to live therapy (Richards & Richardson, 2012).

Such developments are promising, stem from the utilization of new technologies, empirical evidence, and theoretical frameworks, and help address the fact that traditional therapies, though effective, do not work for everyone. Depression is common and debilitating. However, improved and acceptable treatments that will add to our current toolbox of effective interventions can only stem from further developments in basic psychological science that more clearly map the etiological and maintenance risk factors in depression and further our understanding of the characteristics of people who are most vulnerable to the effects of this category of psychological difficulties.

References

Agelink, M. W., Boz, C., Ullrich, H., & Andrich, J. (2002). Relationship between major depression and heart rate variability: Clinical consequences and implications for antidepressive treatment. *Psychiatry Research, 113*, 139–149.

Alloy, L. B., Abramson, L. Y., Hogan, M. E., Whitehouse, W. G., Rose, D. T., Robinson, M. S., … Lapkin, J. B. (2000). The temple-wisconsin cognitive vulnerability to depression project: Lifetime history of axis I psychopathology in individuals at high and low cognitive risk for depression. *Journal of Abnormal Psychology, 109*, 403–418.

Alloy, L. B., Abramson, L. Y., Walshaw, P. D., & Neeren, A. M. (2006). Cognitive vulnerability to unipolar and bipolar mood disorders. *Journal of Social and Clinical Psychology, 25*, 726–754.

American Psychiatric Association (APA). (2013). *Diagnostic and statistical manual of mental disorders* (5th ed.). Washington, DC: Author.

Armstrong, T., & Olatunji, B. O. (2012). Eye tracking of attention in the affective disorders: A meta-analytic review and synthesis. *Clinical Psychology Review, 32*, 704–723.

Bebbington, P. E. (1998). Sex and depression. *Psychological Medicine, 28*, 1–8.

Beck, A. T. (Ed.). (1979). *Cognitive therapy of depression*. New York, NY: Guilford press.

Beck, J. S. (1995). *Cognitive therapy: Basics and beyond*. New York, NY: Guilford Press.

Beevers, C. G., Clasen, P. C., Enock, P. M., & Schnyer, D. M. (2015). Attention bias modification for major depressive disorder: Effects on attention bias, resting state connectivity, and symptom change. *Journal of Abnormal Psychology, 124*, 463.

Brown, G. W. (2002). Social roles, context and evolution in the origins of depression. *Journal of Health and Social Behavior, 43*, 255–276.

Costello, J. E., Erkanli, A., & Angold, A. (2006). Is there an epidemic of child or adolescent depression? *Journal of Child Psychology and Psychiatry, 47*, 1263–1271.

Cristea, I. A., Kok, R. N., & Cuijpers, P. (2015). Efficacy of cognitive bias modification interventions in anxiety and depression: Meta-analysis. *The British Journal of Psychiatry, 206*, 7–16.

Carney, R. M., Blumenthal, J. A., Stein, P. K., Watkins, L., Catellier, D., Berkman, L. F., … & Freedland, K. E. (2001). Depression, heart rate variability, and acute myocardial infarction. *Circulation, 104*(17), 2024–2028.

De Raedt, R., & Koster, E. H. (2010). Understanding vulnerability for depression from a cognitive neuroscience perspective: A reappraisal of attentional factors and a new conceptual framework. *Cognitive, Affective, & Behavioral Neuroscience, 10*, 50–70.

Dekker, M. C., Ferdinand, R. F., Van Lang, N. D., Bongers, I. L., Van Der Ende, J., & Verhulst, F. C. (2007). Developmental trajectories of depressive symptoms from early childhood to late adolescence: Gender differences and adult outcome. *Journal of Child Psychology and Psychiatry, 48*, 657–666.

Dimidjian, S., Hollon, S. D., Dobson, K. S., Schmaling, K. B., Kohlenberg, R. J., Addis, M. E., ... Atkins, D. C. (2006). Randomized trial of behavioral activation, cognitive therapy, and antidepressant medication in the acute treatment of adults with major depression. *Journal of Consulting and Clinical Psychology, 74*, 658–670.

Dimidjian, S., Martell, C. R., Addis, M. E., & Herman-Dunn, R. (2008). Behavioral activation for depression. In D. Barlow (Ed.), *Clinical handbook of psychological disorders*. New York, NY: Guildford Press.

Eells, T. D. (Ed.). (2007). *Handbook of psychotherapy case formulation*. New York, NY: Guilford Press.

Ellis, A. (1957). Rational psychotherapy and individual psychology. *Journal of Individual Psychology, 13*, 38–44.

Everaert, J., Koster, E. H., & Derakshan, N. (2012). The combined cognitive bias hypothesis in depression. *Clinical Psychology Review, 32*, 413–424.

Ferster, C. B. (1981). A functional analysis of behavior therapy. In *Behavior therapy for depression: Present status and future directions* (pp. 181–196). London: Academic Press.

Goldstein, B. L., & Klein, D. N. (2014). A review of selected candidate endophenotypes for depression. *Clinical Psychology Review, 34*(5), 417–427.

Gottesman, I. I., & Gould, T. D. (2003). The endophenotype concept in psychiatry: Etymology and strategic intentions. *American Journal of Psychiatry, 160*, 636–645.

Hankin, B. L., & Abramson, L. Y. (2001). Development of gender differences in depression: An elaborated cognitive vulnerability–transactional stress theory. *Psychological Bulletin, 127*, 773.

Hawley, L. L., Ho, M. H. R., Zuroff, D. C., & Blatt, S. J. (2006). The relationship of perfectionism, depression, and therapeutic alliance during treatment for depression: Latent difference score analysis. *Journal of Consulting and Clinical Psychology, 74*, 930–942.

Hawley, L. L., Padesky, C. A., Hollon, S. D., Mancuso, E., Laposa, J. M., Brozina, K., & Segal, Z. V. (2017). Cognitive-behavioral therapy for depression using mind over mood: CBT skill use and differential symptom alleviation. *Behavior Therapy, 48*(1), 29–44.

Hopko, D. R., Lejuez, C. W., Lepage, J. P., Hopko, S. D., & McNeil, D. W. (2003). A brief behavioral activation treatment for depression: A randomized pilot trial within an inpatient psychiatric hospital. *Behavior Modification, 27*(4), 458–469.

Ingram, R. E. (1984). Toward an information-processing analysis of depression. *Cognitive Therapy and Research, 8*, 443–477.

Ingram, R. E., Miranda, J., & Segal, Z. V. (1998). *Cognitive vulnerability to depression*. New York, NY: Guilford Press.

Joormann, J., Waugh, C. E., & Gotlib, I. H. (2015). Cognitive bias modification for interpretation in major depression: Effects on memory and stress reactivity. *Clinical Psychological Science, 3*, 126–139.

Joormann, J., Yoon, K. L., & Zetsche, U. (2007). Cognitive inhibition in depression. *Applied and Preventive Psychology, 12*, 128–139.

Kazantzis, N., Fairburn, C. G., Padesky, C. A., Reinecke, M., & Teesson, M. (2014). Unresolved issues regarding the research and practice of cognitive behavior therapy: The case of guided discovery using Socratic questioning. *Behaviour Change, 31*, 1–17.

Kendler, K. S., Gardner, C. O., Neale, M. C., Aggen, S., Heath, A., Colodro-Conde, L., ... Gillespie, N. A. (2019). Shared and specific genetic risk factors for lifetime major depression, depressive symptoms and neuroticism in three population-based twin samples. *Psychological Medicine, 49*(16), 2745–2753.

Kendler, K. S., Gatz, M., Gardner, C. O., & Pedersen, N. L. (2006). Personality and major depression: A Swedish longitudinal, population-based twin study. *Archives of General Psychiatry, 63*(10), 1113–1120.

Kendler, K. S., Kuhn, J., & Prescott, C. A. (2004). The interrelationship of neuroticism, sex, and stressful life events in the prediction of episodes of major depression. *American Journal of Psychiatry, 161*, 631–636.

Kendler, K. S., & Myers, J. (2010). The genetic and environmental relationship between major depression and the five-factor model of personality. *Psychological Medicine, 40*, 801–806.

Koster, E. H., De Raedt, R., Leyman, L., & De Lissnyder, E. (2010). Mood-congruent attention and memory bias in dysphoria: Exploring the coherence among information-processing biases. *Behaviour Research and Therapy, 48*, 219–225.

Kujawa, A. J., Torpey, D., Kim, J., Hajcak, G., Rose, S., Gotlib, I. H., & Klein, D. N. (2011). Attentional biases for emotional faces in young children of mothers with chronic or recurrent depression. *Journal of Abnormal Child Psychology, 39*, 125–135.

Lejuez, C. W., Hopko, D. R., & Hopko, S. D. (2001). A brief behavioral activation treatment for depression: Treatment manual. *Behavior Modification, 25*(2), 255–286.

Lim, C. R., Barlas, J., & Ho, R. C. M. (2018). The effects of temperament on depression according to the schema model: A scoping review. *International Journal of Environmental Research and Public Health, 15*(6), 1231.

MacLeod, C., & Mathews, A. (2012). Cognitive bias modification approaches to anxiety. *Annual Review of Clinical Psychology, 8*, 189–217.

Neophytou, K. (2019). *Attention bias modification treatment for social anxiety: Avoidance or exposure to threatening faces*. Unpublished dissertation, University of Cyprus.

Nolen, H. S., Wisco, E., & Lyubomirsky, S. (2008). Rethinking rumination. *Perspectives on Psychological Science, 3*, 400–424.

Nolen-Hoeksema, S. (1987). Sex differences in unipolar depression: Evidence and theory. *Psychological Bulletin, 101*, 259.

Nolen-Hoeksema, S. (1991). Responses to depression and their effects on the duration of depressive episodes. *Journal of Abnormal Psychology, 100*, 569.

Padesky, C. A., & Greenberger, D. (2012). *Clinician's guide to mind over mood*. New York, NY: Guilford Press.

Palsson, S., & Skoog, I. (1997). The epidemiology of affective disorders in the elderly: A review. *International Clinical Psychopharmacology, 12*, S3–S13.

Panayiotou, G. (2018). Alexithymia as a core trait in psychosomatic and other psychological disorders. In C. Charis & G. Panayiotou (Eds.), *Somatoform and other psychosomatic disorders* (pp. 89–106). Cham: Springer.

Panayiotou, G., Brown, R., & Vrana, S. R. (2007). Emotional dimensions as determinants of self-focused attention. *Cognition and Emotion, 21*, 982–998.

Panayiotou, G., Karekla, M., & Leonidou, C. (2017). Coping through avoidance may explain gender disparities in anxiety. *Journal of Contextual Behavioral Science, 6*(2), 215–220.

Panayiotou, G., Karekla, M., & Mete, I. (2014). Dispositional coping in individuals with anxiety disorder symptomatology: Avoidance predicts distress. *Journal of Contextual Behavioral Science, 3*, 314–321.

Panayiotou, G., & Kokkinos, C. M. (2006). Self-consciousness and psychological distress: A study using the Greek SCS. *Personality and Individual Differences, 41*, 83–93.

Panayiotou, G., Panteli, M., & Vlemincx, E. (2018). Processing emotions in alexithymia: A systematic review of physiological markers. In O. Luminet, R. M. Bagby, & G. J. Taylor (Eds.), *Alexithymia: Advances in research, theory, and clinical practice*. Cambridge: Cambridge University Press.

Panayiotou, G., Panteli, M., & Vlemincx, E. (2019). Adaptive and maladaptive emotion processing and regulation, and the case of alexithymia. *Cognition and Emotion*, 1–12.

Panayiotou, G., & Papageorgiou, M. (2007). Depressed mood: The role of negative thoughts, self-consciousness, and sex role stereotypes. *International Journal of Psychology, 42*, 289–296.

Panayiotou, G., & Vrana, S. R. (1998). Effect of self-focused attention on the startle reflex, heart rate, and memory performance among socially anxious and nonanxious individuals. *Psychophysiology, 35*, 328–336.

Peckham, A. D., McHugh, R. K., & Otto, M. W. (2010). A meta-analysis of the magnitude of biased attention in depression. *Depression and Anxiety, 27*, 1135–1142.

Piccinelli, M., & Wilkinson, G. (2000). Gender differences in depression: Critical review. *The British Journal of Psychiatry, 177*, 486–492.

Porges, S. W. (2001). The polyvagal theory: Phylogenetic substrates of a social nervous system. *International Journal of Psychophysiology, 42*, 123–146.

Radloff, L. (1975). Sex differences in depression. *Sex Roles, 1*, 249–265.

Richards, D., & Richardson, T. (2012). Computer-based psychological treatments for depression: A systematic review and meta-analysis. *Clinical Psychology Review, 32*, 329–342.

Sauer-Zavala, S., Gutner, C. A., Farchione, T. J., Boettcher, H. T., Bullis, J. R., & Barlow, D. H. (2017). Current definitions of "trans-diagnostic" in treatment development: A search for consensus. *Behavior Therapy, 48*, 128–138.

Schiweck, C., Piette, D., Berckmans, D., Claes, S., & Vrieze, E. (2019). Heart rate and high frequency heart rate variability during stress as biomarker for clinical depression. A systematic review. *Psychological Medicine, 49*, 200–211.

Theodorou, C. (2020). *Enhancement of emotion regulation skills in vulnerable adolescents due to the existence of addictions or psychopathology in the family*. Unpublished Dissertation, University of Cyprus.

Whiteford, H. A., Harris, M. G., McKeon, G., Baxter, A., Pennell, C., Barendregt, J. J., & Wang, J. (2013). Estimating remission from untreated major depression: A systematic review and meta-analysis. *Psychological Medicine, 43*, 1569–1585.

Williams, A. D., O'Moore, K., Blackwell, S. E., Smith, J., Holmes, E. A., & Andrews, G. (2015). Positive imagery cognitive bias modification (CBM) and internet-based cognitive behavioral therapy (iCBT): A randomized controlled trial. *Journal of Affective Disorders, 178*, 131–141.

Williams, J. M. G., Barnhofer, T., Crane, C., Herman, D., Raes, F., Watkins, E., & Dalgleish, T. (2007). Autobiographical memory specificity and emotional disorder. *Psychological Bulletin, 133*, 122.

Williams, K. M., Iacono, W. G., & Remick, R. A. (1985). Electrodermal activity among subtypes of depression. *Biological Psychiatry, 20*, 158–162.

Williams, L. M. (2016). Precision psychiatry: A neural circuit taxonomy for depression and anxiety. *The Lancet Psychiatry, 3*, 472–480.

Wisco, B. E., & Nolen-Hoeksema, S. (2010). Interpretation bias and depressive symptoms: The role of self-relevance. *Behaviour Research and Therapy, 48*, 1113–1122.

Wittchen, H. U., Jacobi, F., Rehm, J., Gustavsson, A., Svensson, M., Jönsson, B., ... Fratiglioni, L. (2011). The size and burden of mental disorders and other disorders of the brain in Europe 2010. *European Neuropsychopharmacology, 21*, 655–679.

World Health Organization. (2020). Retrieved from https://www.who.int/news-room/fact-sheets/detail/depression

Wray, N. R., Ripke, S., Mattheisen, M., Trzaskowski, M., Byrne, E. M., Abdellaoui, A., ... Bacanu, S. A. (2018). Genome-wide association analyses identify 44 risk variants and refine the genetic architecture of major depression. *Nature Genetics, 50*, 668–681.

Yang, W., Ding, Z., Dai, T., Peng, F., & Zhang, J. X. (2015). Attention bias modification training in individuals with depressive symptoms: A randomized controlled trial. *Journal of Behavior Therapy and Experimental Psychiatry, 49*, 101–111.

Chapter 9
The Acceptance and Commitment Therapy Perspective: Case Conceptualization and Treatment of Depression in Cancer

Marianna Zacharia and Maria Karekla

Contents

9.1   Acceptance and Commitment Therapy Applied to Cancer Care

Acceptance and commitment therapy (ACT) is a theory-driven behavioral approach rooted in functional contextualism and relational frame theory (RFT; Hayes, Strosahl, & Wilson, 2012). In contrast to cognitive behavioral therapy (CBT), which aims to alter the form, content, and frequency of maladaptive thoughts (Beck, 2011), ACT aims to influence the individual's relationship with thoughts so as to decrease their impact on behavior (Hayes, Strosahl, & Wilson, 2012). This objective is achieved by analyzing the experience of the individual within a context of personal values, encouraging acceptance of one's thoughts, emotions, and bodily sensations and committing to behavior change consistent with one's values (Hayes & Lillis, 2012). In doing so, ACT increases psychological flexibility, which is defined as the capacity to be more consciously in contact with the present moment and the ability to adapt to internal or external situational demands in order to pursue long-term values (Karekla, Karademas, & Gloster, 2019; Kashdan & Rottenberg, 2010). Psychological inflexibility (the opposite of psychological flexibility) is regarded as the primary cause of psychopathology (Hayes, Luoma, Bond, Masuda, & Lillis, 2006).

M. Zacharia · M. Karekla (✉)
ACThealthy Laboratory, Department of Psychology, University of Cyprus, Nicosia, Cyprus
e-mail: zacharia.marianna@ucy.ac.cy; mkarekla@ucy.ac.cy

© Springer Nature Switzerland AG 2021
C. Charis, G. Panayiotou (eds.), *Depression Conceptualization and Treatment*,
https://doi.org/10.1007/978-3-030-68932-2_9

Psychological flexibility is established through six interrelated processes that together form the psychological flexibility model (and its inverse the psychological inflexibility model): experiential acceptance (vs. experiential avoidance), cognitive defusion (vs. cognitive fusion), contact with the present moment (vs. dominance of the conceptualized past and future), self as context (vs. attachment to a conceptualized self), values clarification (vs. confusion about what is important for the person, behavior incongruous to one's values), and committed action (vs. inaction, impulsivity, or persistent avoidant behaving; Hayes, Strosahl, & Wilson, 2012). These components are hypothesized to constitute mechanisms of change via which ACT exerts its effects (Forman, Herbert, Moitra, Yeomans, & Geller, 2007; Karekla, Karademas, & Gloster, 2019).

Experiential avoidance is the attempt to modify or control situational sensitivity, frequency, and form of private events (Hayes, Wilson, Gifford, Follette, & Strosahl, 1996; Monestès et al., 2018). For dealing with experiential avoidance, ACT proposes active acceptance of all private events (i.e., thoughts, emotions, bodily sensations, memories) without attempting to alter their form, frequency, or content (Hayes et al., 2006). This must not be confused with giving up or tolerating negative experiences. Cancer patients are frequently told to adopt a fighting spirit attitude, which may in fact involve experiential avoidance of feelings of hopelessness and fear of death (Hulbert-Williams, Storey, & Wilson, 2015). Instead, via acceptance, patients are supported to acknowledge and experience all aspects of their present situation irrespective of social desirability and pressures (Hulbert-Williams et al., 2015; Karekla, Zacharia, & Koushiou, 2018).

Cognitive fusion is "the tendency for behavior to be overly regulated and influenced by cognition" (Gillanders et al., 2014, p. 84). Cognitive fusion consists of the believability of thoughts, dominance of thoughts over characteristics of the experience, struggle in taking into consideration alternative viewpoints on cognitions, and struggling with attempts to control thoughts (Gillanders et al., 2014). This happens when individuals become attached to content instead of the function of cognitions (Luoma & Hayes, 2003). For instance, a patient who smokes may be fused with the thought that he/she has caused his/her cancer and may spend a lot of time ruminating regarding the unhealthy choices he/she has made, which can cause more distress and helplessness (Hooper, Dack, Karekla, Niyazi, & McHugh, 2018; Hulbert-Williams et al., 2015). Cognitive defusion is the opposite of cognitive fusion and refers to the ability to observe inner private events from a distance so as to gradually understand that they are not rules or facts that govern behavior but ways an individual represents the world, and may be ineffective under certain conditions (Gillanders, Sinclair, MacLean, & Jardine, 2015; Karekla et al., 2020).

Contact with the present moment decreases when a person engages in experiential avoidance and cognitive fusion. The conceptualized past and future take control of the present to impact how behavior is regulated (Theofanous, Ioannou, Zacharia, Georgiou, & Karekla, 2020). ACT promotes an open experience of the external and internal events whether perceived as good or bad in the present and promotes present-moment awareness or mindfulness (Biglan, Hayes, & Pistorello, 2008). For cancer patients, rather than focusing exclusively on positive, fighting spirit attitudes, patients must be allowed to encounter and articulate all aspects, including distressing ones (Hulbert-Williams et al., 2015). With ACT, emphasis is on the present instead of being stuck in the past ("how I used to be, or things used to be") or future ("I will never feel the same again").

Moreover, individuals with cancer may fail to differentiate between their cognitive and emotional experiences as being separate from their identity/self and may result in cyclical cognitive appraisals of the self as being ineffectual or that the situation is hopeless (Karekla et al., 2018). When a person becomes "fused" with such attributes (e.g., "I am a cancer patient"), the way the person views himself/herself becomes narrow leading to inflexible behavioral patterns based on these conceptualizations ("self as content"; Luoma, Hayes, & Walser, 2007). ACT promotes the ability to be consistently mindful of feelings, cognitions, and other internal states (*process*) and notice that these private events are different from the experiencing self (*context*; Hayes et al., 2006). When a person is fused with one's experiences, this may restrict other occurrences and aspects of the self to be expressed simultaneously. For example, "I am a cancer patient" may interfere with "I am a good wife" (Karekla et al., 2018), which may cause an attachment to a damaged conceptualized self and in turn impact behavior (e.g., medical treatment adherence; Karekla & Constantinou, 2010).

Values are intrinsic reinforcers, which provide a chosen direction for one's behaviors and actions despite obstacles faced (Wilson & DuFrene, 2009; Wilson & Sandoz, 2008). They are also described as long-term desired qualities of life that cannot be attained as an object (Hayes et al., 2006, p. 8). When values are set aside and emphasis is placed on achieving immediate goals of feeling or looking good, being right, etc., individuals lose contact with what they find meaningful in life (Hayes et al., 2006). For cancer patients, values clarity may help integrating the experience of cancer into their autobiography and sense of self (Fashler, Weinrib, Azam, & Katz, 2018) and their belief system (Karekla & Constantinou, 2010).

In ACT, living a values-consistent life (i.e., committed action—taking action in line with valued directions) is strongly encouraged. Values may be lost or become overshadowed by the problems related to the disease and due to cognitive fusion (Hayes et al., 2006). It is thus vital to set health-related and other goals in line with personal values (i.e., "I will walk for 15 min per day (goal) so as to be healthy (value)" instead of "I have to or must walk for 15 min"; Karekla et al., 2018). Then, patients commit to specific actions to achieve these valued goals (Hayes et al., 2006; Karekla & Constantinou, 2010). It may be easier for individuals to accept aversive experiences when they are able to find ways to act that are consistent with valued directions (Hayes & Smith, 2005; Karekla, Karademas, & Gloster, 2019). For example, "I am willing to receive chemotherapy and face the side effects (i.e., hair loss, vomiting, nausea, fatigue) as I value my health, I want to live and be able to be there and spend time with my family and friends."

9.2 Why Acceptance and Commitment Therapy for Depression in Cancer Care?

ACT has effectively been used in the management of several psychological and physical health problems, including depression, cancer, and chronic pain (Abad, Bakhtiari, Kashani, & Habibi, 2016; Hayes, Strosahl, & Wilson, 2012; Kyllönen et al., 2018; Najvani, Neshatdoost, Abedi, & Mokarian, 2015; Rost, Wilson, Buchanan, Hildebrandt, & Mutch, 2012; Veehof, Trompetter, Bohlmeijer, & Schreurs, 2016; Wetherell et al., 2011). For example, there is evidence that ACT facilitates lower dropout rates (Karekla, Konstantinou, Ioannou, Kareklas, & Gloster, 2019), is efficacious for treatment-resistant patients (Gloster et al., 2015), and better prepares clients to engage in behavioral change actions, improving thus the efficiency and usability of the intervention (Zhang et al., 2018).

ACT in psychosocial oncology care may be particularly beneficial especially when it comes to dealing with diagnosis and treatment aftermath, such as psychological problems related to anxiety and depression (Páez, Luciano, & Gutiérrez, 2007). While high levels of depression and distress are usually regarded as pathological in clinical practice, what distinguishes ACT from other approaches is its rejection of the "assumption of healthy normality" (Hayes, Strosahl, & Wilson, 2012, p. 5). According to the theory behind ACT, suffering constitutes an inevitable component of human experience and can be addressed by approaching difficult life situations with psychological flexibility (Karekla, Karademas, & Gloster, 2019). This has important ramifications for cancer patients, since a distress response to diagnosis and therapy is usual and expected (Fashler et al., 2018).

Subsequent to a cancer diagnosis and throughout treatment, patients face several concerns and life-changing decisions not just about their therapy but also regarding their future and their families' future (Arman & Rehnsfeldt, 2003; Brooks, Wilson, & Amir, 2011). Some patients may even have to confront their mortality (Zafar, Alexander, Weinfurt, Schulman, & Abernethy, 2009). Cognitive behavioral therapy (CBT) stresses challenging distorted negative thinking and promoting a more balanced viewpoint (Beck, 1993). Nevertheless, negative thoughts concerning prognosis, cancer treatment, and losses in valued life areas like in interpersonal relationships and work are probably not distorted (Fashler et al., 2018). The feelings, thoughts, and bodily sensations individuals with cancer encounter may constitute accurate appraisals of their current situations, and negative illness beliefs and distress may be realistic (Fashler et al., 2018). A person having the thought "I might die" and "my family will be overwhelmed" can be true; thus a cognitive restructuring approach may not be suitable for this situation. Also, insinuations that such experiences are distorted with attempts to alter them may increase the frustration of patients and lead to detrimental psychological outcomes (Karekla, Karademas, & Gloster, 2019).

Specifically, attempts to suppress or avoid negative emotions and thoughts aggravate psychological problems and quality of life in the long term for cancer patients (Hack & Degner, 2004; McCaul et al., 1999; Purdon, 1999). Additionally, adopting a fighting spirit attitude (thinking positive) constitutes a mechanism of cancer patients who attempt to linguistically manage the situation in order to protect others instead of an accurate description of positivity (Wilkinson & Kitzinger, 2000). This happens at the expense of their own mental health as by focusing on adopting a fighting spirit, individuals are at risk of heightened experiences of the negative facets of the cancer experience (Hayes, Strosahl, & Wilson, 2012). That is, in cases where their physical health deteriorates, patients are likely to interpret this as a personal failure and may encounter difficult emotions, such as shame or guilt (Hulbert-Williams et al., 2015).

Conversely, ACT research demonstrates that acceptance of internal experiences (emotions, thoughts, memories, sensations, etc.) in contrast to avoidance is related to lower psychological distress in several cancer populations (Arch et al., 2020; Gregg, 2013; Jensen et al., 2014; Páez et al., 2007; Politi, Enright, & Weihs, 2007; Roesch et al., 2005; Stanton, Danoff-burg, & Huggins, 2002).

ACT is scalable; hence the format, content, number, and length of sessions may differ substantially (Fashler et al., 2018). ACT can be used flexibly according to the needs of the patient population and severity of symptoms. The six processes of ACT can be modeled, taught, and practiced by employing various techniques, including metaphors, experiential exercises, and clinical interactions. The flexible structure of ACT may be particularly suitable for individuals undergoing cancer therapy and encountering adverse psychological effects (e.g., depression). Also, the values clarity work and values-driven committed action emphasis present with novel means so as to achieve current life fulfillment even in the face of difficulties (Fashler et al., 2018). More research is however needed to establish the effectiveness and efficacy of ACT for psychological problems faced by cancer patients and also to examine whether the proposed psychological flexibility model components are the mechanisms via which treatment exerts it effects.

9.3   Case Conceptualization and Treatment of Depression in a Woman with Breast Cancer

To illustrate this approach, we will briefly describe the case of KC, a woman diagnosed with breast cancer who is facing psychological problems (depression) as a result of the cancer diagnosis and medical therapy and for whom an ACT approach was employed. Note that information regarding the case of KC, including the initials, have been disguised in order to protect the client's identity, according to the General Data Protection Regulation (GDPR).

First, we present the case conceptualization (functional behavioral analysis) based on the psychological flexibility model. Then, an ACT-based synthesis of the hypothetical mechanism and a treatment plan are presented. The structure of this case conceptualization and treatment plan is partly based on the following resources: Dr. Karekla's lectures at the University of Cyprus and similar approaches presented in Constantinou and Karekla (2015); Karekla and Constantinou (2010); Luoma, Hayes, and Walser (2017); Persons (2008); Ramnero and Torneke (2008); and Zettle (2007).

9.3.1   Presenting Problem

KC is a 50-year-old woman, who asked for psychological support because of depressed mood and elevated anxiety, following a recent diagnosis of breast cancer followed by a lumpectomy. In particular, she reported feeling overwhelmed and very distressed about the cancer diagnosis. She stated that she has a very limited social support network (only two close friends), from whom however she does not feel support. Regarding family members (two siblings), she expressed that she is the one who is supporting them both emotionally and practically (financially). She expressed that she needed to make all necessary preparations prior to surgery (e.g., purchase of a special bra for use after the lumpectomy surgery of breast cancer, shopping at home, transportation from the hospital to home, driving) by herself and could not expect help from anyone else. She also stated that both of her parents were diagnosed with chronic diseases and she was the one who was exclusively "devoted to their care" until their death (father died 10 years ago and mother died 1 year ago). Additionally, she mentioned that prior to the cancer diagnosis, she was experiencing intense pain and was diagnosed with fibromyalgia. She is employed and her job status has not changed as a result of her diagnosis and treatment.

9.3.2   List of Presenting Problems

First, a comprehensive list based on KC's presenting problems is developed encompassing all the information presented by the client.

Thoughts and Memories

"I do not want to die"; "I am just a cancer patient and nothing else"; "I am responsible for my cancer because I was always stressed"; "Who is to blame and what is to blame?"; "This is my fault"; "Others are to blame for how I am"; "I want to live a better life than the one I am living right now"; "I am tired of maintaining the balance in my family"; "I have not achieved anything in my life. My partners left me"; "I wish I had a partner"; "I have disbelief in the medical system"; "I'll be a burden if I ask the doctors about my concerns"; "I'll be ungrateful if I express my complaints to the doctors"; "Doctors think their work ends in surgery"; "I'd like to tell my doctor that he does not give me the attention that I need"; "I want my doctor to listen to me and I hate it when he tells me that I am strong and I will get over it soon"; "I must be problematic since I do not have a partner"; "I am all alone; nobody understands me"; "I will not be able to find a partner and I am not capable of having a family"; and "My friends only expect me to support them and do not support me in return." She presented with vivid memories of the absence of emotion sharing in her family and the absence of emotional words and actions (e.g., hugs, kisses) and support from her parents or siblings. She also has vivid memories about a parent's preference for her other siblings. Other memories that cause her discomfort are the separation from her previous partners, which she experienced as rejection.

Emotions/Physical Sensations

Confusion, insecurity, sadness, anxiety, fear, disappointment, embarrassment, anger, loneliness, guilt, fatigue, breast pain after surgery, and pain in her joints and muscles (especially on the neck, waist, and buttocks) which existed prior to the breast cancer diagnosis and surgery but increased after surgery and radiotherapy.

Behavior

Stopped engaging in any pleasant activities, rumination (negative persistent thinking), consumes large amounts of food and sweets, isolates at home, avoids social events and communication with her few friends, stays in bed and sleeps instead of doing daily activities and chores, "sitting and waiting" for a partner without seeking to meet anyone, avoids men when they approach her and when they show interest, takes pills daily (painkillers) to reduce physical pain after surgery and radiotherapy (this may extend beyond the period recommended by her doctor), and avoids her manager and most of her colleagues at work.

9.3.3   Predisposing Factors

Predisposing factors are any factors that characterize an individual's vulnerability for developing psychopathology (Laurila, Laakkonen, Laurila, Timo, & Reijo, 2008). Family history of psychological problems may indicate possible genetic predisposition or learning from other family members' behaviors (Nabors, 2020). In this case, the client presented a family history of depressive symptomatology. In particular, one of her parents was chronically depressed after a relative died.

Temperament as a child may constitute another predisposing factor for the development of depressive symptomatology (Wetter & Hankin, 2009; Wilson, DiRago, & Iacono, 2014). KC remembers always experiencing more negative instead of positive emotions. Higher levels of negative emotionality/neuroticism (a tendency to experience negative mental moods) and less stable, lower levels of positive emotionality/extroversion (tendency to experience positive mental moods) are predictors of depression in childhood, adolescence (Wetter & Hankin, 2009), and adulthood (Wilson et al., 2014). Also, negative emotionality in the family, expressed with negative expressions of emotion (verbal and non-verbal), can lead to negative emotions in children and is related to the development of depression (Morris, Silk, Steinberg, Myers, & Robinson, 2007).

Particularly, she mentioned that her parents tended to discourage the expression of emotions, and generally there was a lack of discussion and sharing of their emotions as a family. When she expressed emotions (e.g., anxiety, sadness, joy), she presented that her parents had difficulty listening, understanding, and validating her emotions. Research findings have shown that discouraging the expression of emotions in childhood is an important factor in the development of depression (Silk et al., 2011). Parents who respond to their child's positive feelings in a discouraging manner tend to restrict (e.g., guide the child to calm down), punish (e.g., reprimand or get angry), and prevent (e.g., respond with distress) the expression of positive feelings of their child (Yap, Allen, & Ladouceur, 2008). Thus, children who receive these socialization responses learn to suppress the expression of positive emotions and fail to develop adaptive skills to regulate their emotions (Denham, Mitchell-Copeland, Strandberg, Auerbach, & Blair, 1997).

In addition, it is possible that her parents modeled rumination as a response to stressful situations (Nolen-Hoeksema, 1991). Children of depressed parents tend to use less effective strategies like their parents, for example, more passive and less active strategies to regulate their emotions (Garber, Braafladt, & Zeman, 1991; Silk, Shaw, Skuban, Oland, & Kovacs, 2006). That is, they use passive waiting and constantly focus on the source of their discomfort (rumination), aggression, and withdrawal (Silk et al., 2006).

Various psychosocial factors increase the likelihood of developing depression in women with breast cancer (Hopko, McIndoo, Gawrysiak, & Grassetti, 2014). These include lack of a close and trusting relationship, reduced social support, poor family cohesion and many family conflicts, inappropriate problem-solving skills (e.g., rumination), as well as comorbid chronic conditions such as chronic pain (Deshields, Tibbs, Fan, & Taylor, 2006; Lueboonthavatchai, 2007; Yan et al., 2019; Zabora, BrintzenhofeSzoc, Curbow, Hooker, & Piantadosi, 2001). KC appears to meet all these factors. Also, a previous episode of depression, anxiety, or both increases the likelihood of developing depression in women with breast cancer (Burgess et al., 2005). KC seems to have had a previous depressive episode at around the age of 35, when one of her parents was diagnosed with a chronic disease and she became the primary and sole caretaker. Also, she presents as an individual who has been anxious about numerous life situations.

9.3.4 Precipitating Factors

Precipitating factors are specific events or triggers to the onset of the current psychological difficulty (Laurila et al., 2008). Beyond the role of early experiences, exposure to stressful life events in adulthood seems to be related to the onset of episodes of depression (McLaughlin, Conron, Koenen, & Gilman, 2010). In this case, KC had a number of such stressful life events: loss of important romantic relationships, parents' illness and exclusive devotion to their care, and subsequent death of her parents. Another stressful event is the role she takes as being responsible for the resolution of conflicts between other family members (i.e., two siblings).

The most recent stressful factor that seems to have triggered the onset of depressive mood is the diagnosis of breast cancer. The experience of receiving a breast cancer diagnosis and living with cancer is a stressful life event that can trigger a depressive episode (Kissane, Maj, & Sartorius, 2011; Schotte, Van Den Bossche, De Doncker, Claes, & Cosyns, 2006). Also, depressive symptomatology is more likely to occur when a person is experiencing physical pain, particularly chronic pain (Ciaramella & Poli, 2001; Yan et al., 2019).

9.3.5   Mechanisms of Maintaining the Problem According to the Psychological Flexibility Model

Figure 9.1 shows the psychological flexibility model and the ratings provided for this client, based on conceptualizing cases using ACT by Luoma et al. (2017) and Wilson (2009). For this client, the level of pervasiveness of each of the six components of the psychological inflexibility model was rated on a scale of 1 (limited) to 5 (very extensive) (Luoma et al., 2017). A description of each of the components in relation to this case and how the rating came about follows. The inflexibility aspects will be presented, since these difficulties will be targeted in treatment through the psychological flexibility components.

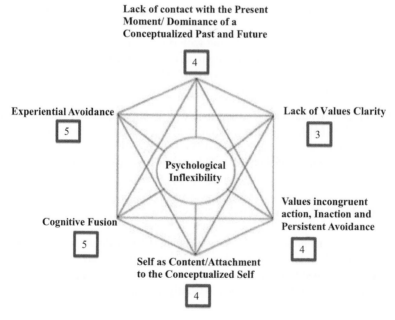

Fig. 9.1 Assessment of the client's skills according to the psychological inflexibility model

Experiential Avoidance

KC presented that she tends to avoid situations that make her experience emotions (calls them "difficult") regarding the diagnosis of cancer (i.e., social interactions, meetings with friends and colleagues). She also avoids expressing negative feelings to friends and colleagues, particularly feelings of anger and resentment. She particularly becomes angry and resentful in situations when her friends and colleagues tell her encouraging words about her health and that she is "lucky" to have caught the cancer early. She also tends to avoid the physical pain she feels by isolating herself at home, taking painkillers and sleeping, and not doing her daily activities/chores. In addition, she consumes large amounts of food and sweets in an attempt to numb negative thoughts and emotions about the cancer prognosis. In her workplace, she avoids almost all of her colleagues and her manager because she sees "pity in their eyes." Regarding romantic relationships, she "sits and waits" without seeking to meet someone, and when it happens that a man approaches her and expresses interest, she avoids him (leaves or does not respond) so as to prevent herself from experiencing rejection.

Internal Emotional Control Strategies Excessive rumination/worry and distraction.

Overt Emotional Control Strategies Eating large amounts of food and sweets, taking painkillers, avoiding work, avoiding social situations/events and conversations, avoiding intimacy with any man who shows interest, staying at home, and sleeping.

Strategies for Avoiding Emotions and Emotional Control Observed During Sessions Changing of subject when difficult issues are discussed (e.g., romantic relationships); focusing exclusively and with rigidity on the negatives; focusing on who or what is to blame and who is right and wrong; focuses on facts and logic to avoid uncomfortable emotions; and exposure to situations that may be meaningful yet may create anxiety.

Overall, experiential avoidance appears to be an important control method pervasive across all of her life areas. If we were to provide a pervasiveness of experiential avoidance rating (see Luoma et al., 2017) on a Likert-type scale of 1 (limited) to 5 (extensive avoidance), this client would probably receive a score of 5.

Cognitive Fusion

During sessions she presented with fusion (being stuck) with the idea that she is not attractive enough to be loved and that she is not going to find a partner. She also presented as attached to her negative thoughts regarding the diagnosis and prognosis of cancer and her self-image. She repeatedly presented the thought that she is the one to blame for her cancer because she was "stressed" and with rigid thinking patterns (i.e., "I am just a cancer patient and nothing else"). KC judges herself very strictly and in an absolute manner ("I have not accomplished anything in my life"), especially when it comes to romantic relationships ("I must be problematic since I do not have a partner"). She sees herself as "a burden" and as "ungrateful" when she has questions or complaints for her doctors. These thoughts she states prevent her from asking questions about the medical treatment and breast reconstruction following the lumpectomy. At times she appeared to get lost in her thinking (missing aspects of conversations). In terms of the extent of KC's cognitive fusion, we rated it similar to experiential avoidance with a score of 5.

Self as Content/Attachment to a Conceptualized Self

Based on the way she talks about herself, KC appears to have a reduced awareness of herself as a "whole" and finds it hard to see herself as something beyond just her thoughts or the difficulties she is facing. She characterizes herself as "problematic" because all the romantic relationships she had to date did not last. She uses words to describe herself as a "victim" regarding the family burdens she undertakes, yet she does not appear willing to not undertake them. The image she has of herself is that she is "a cancer patient and nothing else." She seems to have difficulty seeing beyond her cancer diagnosis and its consequences in her life. Specifically, she seems to equate who she is with the diagnostic label and adopts a helpless stance toward the problem as now determining who she is or will be in the future. The only area where she appears to regard herself as something more than her problems is when it comes to her work, where she expresses that she knows that she is a competent employee and for that she is appreciated by her colleagues. Regarding the level of pervasiveness of attachment to a conceptualized self, we gave her a score of 4.

Lack of Contact with the Present Moment/Dominance of a Conceptualized Past and Future

Often KC appears to "lose herself" in her thoughts about past problems and failures, or a catastrophic future. She is mostly attached to the past, since she often ruminates and presents a continuous thought run-through of searching for "whys" and wanting to attribute blame for her condition and problems. She also thinks that, in the future, she will not be able to find a partner and that she is not capable of having a family. She occasionally focuses on the present when she expresses her present feelings of unhappiness regarding her social and romantic life and the image she has of herself. Regarding the level of pervasiveness of a conceptualized past and future, we gave her a score of 4.

Lack of Values Clarity

Through both the clinical interview and KC's responses to a self-report measure (Valued Living Questionnaire; Wilson, Sandoz, Kitchens, & Roberts, 2010), it emerged that important values for her are close emotional/romantic relationships, family relationships, parenthood, and friendship/social life. From these, she expressed that the most important value is having a close trustworthy romantic relationship. According to her, she often loses contact with this value and avoids meeting a man due to fear of rejection. Other important values for her are work, education, and health/physical care (healthy eating, exercise, sleep). Her education and career progress are the only values where she mostly lives in line with (i.e., her behaviors match her values and the path she would like to be on), whereas for the rest of the values, her behaviors do not align with her values. With the help of the therapist, she was able to identify her valued directions and recognize areas she has not been living in accordance with what is most important to her. As such, in this area we provided a score of 3.

Values-Incongruent Action, Inaction and Persistent Avoidance

KC acts partly in accordance to her values in the professional domain since she is very good at her job and receives positive feedback from her colleagues. She also acts according to the value of being supportive toward her family, providing practical and emotional help to her siblings and their children. She states that this does give her meaning in life, but she also feels overburdened by this or feels like she has to take this on without recognizing that this is a choice she herself makes. KC, however, behaves incongruently to some of her valued domains, such as when she avoids social interactions and meetings with friends and colleagues or avoids experiences that could lead to a romantic relationship. Further, she tries to live a life free of emotional pain which renders her behavioral repertoire to become quite narrow and unsatisfying (i.e., feeling stuck in unsatisfying family roles, lack of meaningful relationships, sleeping to avoid physical and emotional pain). Therefore, regarding the level of inaction and persistently avoidant behavior, we gave her a score of 4.

According to the psychological flexibility/inflexibility model, KC seems to encounter greater difficulty with the processes of experiential avoidance and cognitive fusion, whereas lack of present-moment awareness, attachment to a conceptualized self, and values-incongruent behavior follow. To further examine the mechanisms that maintain her problems, we next examined chains of "ABCs" (Ramnero & Torneke, 2008), where A = Antecedents, B = Behavior, and C = Consequences (see Table 9.1). The aim was to further recognize reinforcement loops that maintain KC's behaviors and depression.

Table 9.1 Indicative ABCs to examine mechanisms that maintain problems

A Activating events/ antecedents	B Behavior	C Consequences (behavioral mechanism/function)
Thinks about her cancer diagnosis/feels sad Experiences physical sensations: pain in the area of the breasts and in the armpit (area of the surgery)	– Rumination ("I am just a cancer patient and nothing else," "I am responsible for my cancer because I was stressed") – Isolates herself—stays at home, stays in bed and sleeps – Does not complete daily activities and chores – Does not go to work – Takes painkillers (maybe beyond the time frame advised by her doctors)	Emotional and physical pain are not exacerbated (negative reinforcement) Immediate emotional relief (positive reinforcement) Friends and colleagues call because they are worried and express their interest—attention and confirmation (positive reinforcement)
Feeling tired, pain in the joints and muscles	– Rumination ("I am just a cancer patient and nothing else," "I must be problematic since I do not have a partner," "Who and what is to blame?") – Stays in bed, sleeps, and avoids daily activities and chores – Takes painkillers (maybe beyond the time frame advised by her doctors)	Reduction of fatigue when she is sleeping (negative reinforcement) Short-term pain reduction (negative reinforcement) Immediate emotional relief (positive reinforcement) Friends and colleagues call because they are worried and express their interest—attention and confirmation (positive reinforcement)
Alone at home Irritable mood, feels lonely, sad, as well as anxious and fearful of the prognosis of cancer Thought: "I do not want to die"	– Consumes large amounts of food and sweets – Avoids all activities that could provide her with pleasure	Satisfaction from the taste of food and sweets (positive reinforcement) Short-term relief from negative emotions (positive reinforcement) Short-term avoidance of negative thoughts (negative reinforcement)
A man approaches her and shows his interest in her	– Avoids the conversation and leaves the place	Avoids the possibility of being rejected (negative reinforcement) Belief: "I must be problematic since I do not have a partner" (positive reinforcement)

(continued)

Table 9.1 (continued)

A Activating events/ antecedents	B Behavior	C Consequences (behavioral mechanism/function)
Colleagues/friends tell her: "You are lucky. Think positive and everything is going to be OK" Emotions: anger, guilt, disappointment, loneliness Thought: "I am all alone; nobody understands me"	– Does not express her emotions to friends/colleagues, leaves the place or hangs up the phone – Avoids social events and communication with colleagues/friends	Avoidance of perceived conflict, which she believes will trigger more negative emotions (negative reinforcement) Short-term avoidance of negative thoughts (negative reinforcement) Short-term relief from negative emotions of anger, guilt, disappointment (positive reinforcement) Others do not become aware of what she would like to hear from them and so continue to behave in the same way (positive reinforcement of her beliefs that "Nobody understands me")
Visits her doctors who try to encourage her by telling her that she is strong and will get over it soon Low mood, guilt, embarrassment, anger Negative thoughts about herself: "I'll be a burden if I ask the doctors about my questions," "I'll be ungrateful if I express my complaints to the doctors," "I must be problematic"	– Remains silent and does not ask doctors the questions she has – Does not express her concerns	Short-term avoidance of negative thoughts about herself (negative reinforcement) Short-term relief from negative emotions (positive reinforcement) Avoidance of the possibility of experiencing rejection from the doctors (negative reinforcement) Continued belief that she is "problematic" (positive reinforcement)

9.3.6 Synthesis of the Hypothesized Mechanism

KC appears to have struggled with depressive feelings in the past, yet her current depressive symptomatology emerged following a breast cancer diagnosis. Her critical stance toward herself, her tendency to avoid her negative emotions through various behaviors, and the intense ruminative thoughts in response to stressful situations may constitute modeling products and ineffectual learning from her parents and her history to date.

According to ACT and the psychological flexibility/inflexibility model, depressive symptomatology and problems exist mainly due to experiential avoidance, cognitive fusion, attachment to the past or foreseeing a catastrophic future (lack of living in the present), and lack of values-congruent behavior. KC tries to control and regulate her emotions through rumination and distraction, eating large amounts of food and sweets, and avoiding social situations and events which she believes may cause her to experience negative emotions. She seeks to control emotional and physical pain by avoiding her job, by staying at home and sleeping, as well as taking painkillers. It seems that through rumination she avoids, in the short term, contact with negative emotions. All these dysfunctional behaviors are reinforced through both positive and negative reinforcement loops that result in the maintenance of these behavioral patterns and exacerbation of depression and lack of contact with any pleasurable or valued activities.

From an early age, she adopted certain dysfunctional behavioral coping and emotion regulation patterns with difficult and distressing situations, thoughts, and emotions, and all these contribute to psychopathogenesis and the maintenance of depressive symptomatology. She presents a rigid and absolute way of thinking and strictly judges herself ("problematic," "ungrateful," "a burden"). She is attached to a conceptualized self and seems to treat herself as a problem that needs to be solved. She is having a hard time seeing herself as something beyond her thoughts, inadequacies, and problems.

She is often not in the present moment, which sustains her depressive symptomatology. She is often ruminating about her failures or traumatic experiences from the past in terms of her romantic relationships ("I have not achieved anything in my life. My partners left me. I wish I had a partner"), which she generalizes to predicting a potential catastrophic future. Specifically, she becomes entangled with thoughts about a disastrous future of loneliness, inability to find a partner, and being incapable of forming a family.

Further, her avoidance behavior with the short-term goals of "being right," "feeling good," protecting the conceptualized self, and avoiding rejection (by a partner or her doctors) prevents her from living in line with her values. When she seeks relief from psychological and physical pain through control and avoidance and when she is attached to her thoughts, she does not act according to her values (e.g., in the areas of romantic relationships, forming her own family, and friendships). The context in which her values function at this stage is limited, but she acts according to some of her values (to be a good sister, a good employee).

The function of her depressive behavior (rumination, staying at home and sleeping instead of going to work, not doing daily activities/chores, not expressing her emotions and thoughts to others, eating large amounts of food particularly sweets) has a double reinforcing role. On the one hand, it acts via negative reinforcement since she avoids pain, negative emotions (especially sadness and loneliness), and perceived conflict (that could bring about more "negative" emotions) and reduces fatigue in the short term. On the other hand, it acts via positive reinforcement since when she stays at home and does not go to work, she receives attention from her friends and colleagues who are worried and call her expressing their interest and experiences temporary emotional relief. Also, when she takes painkillers and stays in bed ruminating, her belief that she is "problematic" is positively reinforced. By eating sweets, she receives satisfaction from the taste of food. As a consequence of her lack of expressing emotions and thoughts, individuals do not understand her, which reinforces her belief that nobody understands her (positive reinforcement).

These functions maintain her depressive symptomatology. In the long term, staying at home, sleeping, and not doing pleasant and meaningful activities lead to more physical pain, more rumination about herself, and difficult emotions.

9.3.7 Strengths That Can Aid the Intervention

KC reached for help on her own, recognizing the difficulties she is facing and presenting as motivated to make changes in her life. She has a stable job which presents her with satisfaction and economic means and from where she has established relationships with colleagues and her manager. She has a few friends and some family members that can provide social support. She also seems to have a good medical team that support her and provide her with state-of-the-art treatments. Her cancer prognosis is also good.

9.3.8 External Barriers or Obstacles to the Intervention

Although KC does have some friends and family members, the extent that they can provide meaningful social support is questionable and needs to be further explored. Thus, a lack of a stable social support network or previously learned patterns of interaction with her family and friends may act as a barrier to the intervention. KC's health prognosis is good; however, treatments and possible side effects and complications need to be considered.

9.4 Treatment Plan

Based on the functional analysis and case formulation above, the treatment plan follows an ACT perspective and utilizes the psychological flexibility model to propose intervention targets. As such, the ultimate goal of therapy is to achieve functional and quality living, where the client is able to become fully functional in her life, living in accordance to her values and demonstrating psychological flexibility in emotional, cognitive, and behavioral areas. It goes without saying that all interventions are couched within a good therapeutic relationship based on empathy, trust, authenticity, unconditional positive regard, and acceptance is paramount. The therapy process will be a continuous loop of assessment, treatment, evaluation of outcome, and back again as needed.

Treatment will begin by targeting the psychological flexibility processes that show more weakness, since it is expected that this will have a greater impact on the clients' functionality and quality of life (Hayes, Strosahl, & Wilson, 1999). However, given that the processes are hypothesized to be linked, some concepts will overlap, or some of the exercises may function to target more than one model component. In the case of KC, we suggest starting with cognitive defusion and experiential acceptance as the first intervention targets while bringing in concepts of self as context, present-moment awareness, and values-driven behaviors in the process. In order to reduce experiential control and to encourage acceptance, "creative hopelessness" will be introduced to highlight the futility of efforts to control depression and physical and emotional pain. ACT utilizes metaphors and experiential exercises to instigate learning and experientially (vs. verbally) demonstrate concepts, so in this case metaphors like the "Person in the Hole" can be used. The pervasiveness and normalcy of experiential control will be discussed in order to reduce her self-blaming and validate her struggles with depression and pain (Zettle, 2007). Next, emphasis will be placed on the futility and the cost of experiential control through exercises drawn from KC's experiences (e.g., "Don't think about ..." and "Falling in Love Metaphor"). There will be a focus on willingness as an alternative to experiential control (e.g., "Carrying Your Depression Exercise"; Zettle, 2007). Active acceptance of all private events (thoughts, emotions, physical sensations, memories) will be promoted without attempting to change their form, frequency, or content (Hayes et al., 2006). Some exercises that can be used for this purpose are "Physicalizing Exercise" for accepting unwanted feelings and "Sitting with Feelings Exercise" for accepting feelings, related thoughts, bodily sensations, and memories.

At the same time, emphasis will be placed on cognitive defusion. This involves some psychoeducation of how emotions and thoughts evolved in humans and normalizing that thoughts and emotions are not by their nature problematic, and all have a function and a role to play in our lives. Experientially we will present when thoughts and emotions become problematic, when we are trapped in them and give them all of our attention by holding the content of our thoughts as literally true and then believing that the only way we can function is by getting rid of them. The goal is to keep some distance from her thoughts, make some space for her thoughts to exist and to be able to see her thoughts as they are, as thoughts and nothing more. Techniques and exercises that can be used are "The mind in the third person" technique; the exercise "Your mind is not your friend" so as to promote observing the process of self-evaluation rather than responding to the content and the self-evaluation; the technique "Thank your Mind" which can be used to recognize the troublesome content of her mind and help her understand that her mind is functioning fine and that efforts to control her mind (i.e., stop or change the content, frequency, and form of her thoughts) are ineffective; and the "Milk, Milk, Milk" exercise which can be used to focus on distinguishing self-evaluations from descriptions (self-evaluations versus descriptions) and encourage her to describe her thinking (e.g., "Now I have the thought that ... I am problematic"). In addition, the exercise "Why, why, why" and the "Flat Tire Metaphor" can be used to defuse reason giving, that is, to emphasize how rumination can prevent her from living her life according to her values.

Similarly, and through this process, self as context will be promoted. The aim is for the client to start to experience herself as an arena of experiences, including the experience of cancer, and as a safe place from which she can engage in exposure. The "observing self" will be identified, and metaphors and experiential exercises will be used to become aware of, understand, and distinguish the "observing self" from the "thinking self" (e.g., utilize the "Chessboard Metaphor" or "Furniture in the House Metaphor"). The therapeutic relationship will be used to model the processes of ACT in session, to reduce attachment to the conceptualized self and promote self as context.

At the same time, contact with the present moment will be fostered, i.e., flexible and present-moment awareness to current situations and events (internal and external). Mindfulness techniques will be utilized to learn to live in the here and now and to be able to utilize the senses to return to the present moment when the mind starts to wonder and become entangled with thoughts and feelings. The aim is to experience external events in the environment and internal events as they occur without being absorbed by thoughts about the past or the future. Mindfulness will promote relating to internal private events in a nonevaluative manner. Exercises will be done both in session and outside therapy, such as mindful eating and breathing, "Soldiers in the Parade," "Sky Metaphor," "Leaves on a Stream," and "Watching the Mind-Train." There will also be encouragement to perform daily activities with mindfulness (e.g., to eat, drink, and walk mindfully). There will be no focus on "fighting spirit attitudes" but instead on being able to experience and express all her feelings, thoughts, and physical sensations in the here and now, including unpleasant ones.

Further identification of important values and areas which give her meaning will follow, by identifying the things for which she chooses to live for. This process will help identify pleasurable and reinforcement providing activities for KC. Committed actions directed toward her values even when experiencing physical pain, negative thoughts, and negative emotions (e.g., loneliness, grief, guilt, embarrassment, anger, etc.) will be promoted. In the long term, the treatment will aim to empower her by improving her self-image and helping her develop a more compassionate attitude toward herself.

Regarding the values work, values will be explored as long-term desirable life directions, which cannot be achieved as objects and "can be instantiated moment by moment" (Hayes et al., 2006, p. 8). The difference between values and goals will be highlighted. In the initial assessment of values, the following exercises can be used: "Which hero do you admire?"; "Revisit the wishes of your childhood"; "Epitaph Exercise"; and "What do you want your life to stand for?". Relevant goals for each value can be discussed and identified. KC will be encouraged to choose small and achievable committed valued actions at each time and for each day. There will be a discussion that certain goals are more long-term and various graduated steps may be required. Behavior activation techniques will also be utilized here.

A modest level of action will be set and then gradually KC can progress to more ambitious levels of action. In addition, obstacles and barriers to commitment will be managed in collaboration with the client (Zettle, 2007). Adverse physical sensations (e.g., pain), thoughts, and emotions that are obstacles to making a committed action will be discussed, and ways of responding to these unwanted experiential barriers will be explored. The "Passengers on the Bus Metaphor" and the "Swamp Exercise" ("Are you willing to go through the swamp and get dirty for what gives you meaning in life, for your values?") will be used. The practice of ACT techniques in contexts outside treatment will be encouraged.

Finally, for any areas where we identify lack of skills (e.g., communication and expression of emotions and needs), skills training, exercises, and practice will be carried out (e.g., assertiveness training, saying "no," social and relationship skills, etc.). As aforementioned, a continuous evaluation and monitoring of outcomes will be taking place, so at any point we identify areas where additional skills or modifications are needed; these will be carried out accordingly with the aim of achieving psychological flexibility and valued-based living.

9.4.1 Termination and Relapse Prevention

Termination will be decided in accordance with KC ensuring that she will continue to apply and further develop what she has learned and achieved in therapy. Various techniques that can act as reminders and prompts can be introduced, such as the prompt card proposed by Zettle (2007). In this exercise, one side of the prompt card includes the FEAR acronym addressing obstacles to willingness (Fusion with thoughts, Evaluation, Avoidance, and Reason giving for experiences) and the other side includes the ACT acronym (Accept your reactions and be present, Choose a valued direction, Take action).

For relapse prevention, the external (i.e., situations) and internal (i.e., thoughts, emotions, physical sensations) warning signs likely to trigger relapse will be addressed. Then, in collaboration with KC, an individualized relapse prevention plan will be developed that will include ways in which she can support herself and ways she can get support from her family or friends. Here too as in all other aspects of the intervention, KC will be guided and encouraged to identify, discuss, and use her strengths to enhance her psychological flexibility and resilience.

9.4.2 Assessment of Progress

Only a few sessions have been done with KC thus far. Progress noted so far include that she is now able to see herself through another context, that of a successful woman in the professional domain. Also, she seems to be able to see other aspects of herself now, such as being intelligent, being a good sister, and being a good friend. She now articulates goals and values for her life that are heartfelt and meaningful (romantic relationships, health, friendship). Additionally, she started engaging in actions according to the value of being physically and psychologically healthy. For example, in addition to starting therapy and being committed in the therapeutic process, she began personal training and is more willing and has started to expose herself in situations that are in line with valued life directions (i.e., meet with friends and express her thoughts and feelings to them).

The evaluation of progress and intervention effectiveness will be continuously carried out in collaboration with KC and particularly in evaluating goals achieved in accordance with valued areas. Additionally, progress will be evaluated through clinical observation by the therapist within the sessions and the way the client herself regards her progress or demonstrates changes in her life. The following self-report scales can also be used to evaluate progress: Hospital Anxiety and Depression Scale (Zigmond & Snaith, 1983), Greek Psychological Inflexibility in Pain Scale (Vasiliou, Michaelides, Kasinopoulos, & Karekla, 2019), Greek Acceptance and Action Questionnaire–II (Karekla & Michaelides, 2017), Greek–Cognitive Fusion Questionnaire (Zacharia, Ioannou, Theofanous, Vasiliou, & Karekla, 2021), Cognitive and Affective Mindfulness Scale Revised (Feldman, Hayes, Kumar, Greeson, & Laurenceau, 2007), Valued Living Questionnaire (Wilson et al., 2010), and the Psyflex (English version: Firsching et al., 2018; Greek version: Paraskeva-Siamata, Spyridou, Gloster, & Karekla, 2018). Additionally, risk assessment will be performed at frequent time intervals and managed if necessary. Ideally, it would be good to corroborate progress with more objective assessments and maybe in the reports of others in her life. The overall prognosis appears good for KC.

In conclusion, this chapter illustrated the acceptance and commitment therapy approach to case conceptualization and treatment plan for a client presenting with depression following a diagnosis and lumpectomy for breast cancer. The ACT approach appears to be an effective therapeutic approach transdiagnostically for psychopathological conditions, including depression, with outcomes (both functionality and quality of life improvements and depressive symptom reductions) and effect sizes paralleling that of other empirically supported interventions (Twohig & Levin, 2017). ACT via its psychological flexibility model is malleable and can be easily adapted to the specific needs of real-life client cases who often present with a multitude of problems and comorbidities, such as the case illustrated here.

References

Abad, A. N. S., Bakhtiari, M., Kashani, F. L., & Habibi, M. (2016). The comparison of effectiveness of treatment based on acceptance and commitment with cognitive-behavioral therapy in reduction of stress and anxiety in cancer patients. *International Journal of Cancer Research and Prevention, 9*(3), 229–246.

Arch, J. J., Fishbein, J. N., Ferris, M. C., Mitchell, J. L., Levin, M. E., Slivjak, E. T., … Kutner, J. S. (2020). Acceptability, feasibility, and efficacy potential of a multimodal acceptance and commitment therapy intervention to address psychosocial and advance care planning needs among anxious and depressed adults with metastatic cancer. *Journal of Palliative Medicine, 23*, 1380. https://doi.org/10.1089/jpm.2019.0398

Arman, M., & Rehnsfeldt, A. (2003). The hidden suffering among breast cancer patients: A qualitative metasynthesis. *Qualitative Health Research, 13*(4), 510–527. https://doi.org/10.117 7/2F1049732302250721

Beck, A. T. (1993). Cognitive therapy: Past, present, and future: Recent developments in cognitive and constructivist psychotherapies. *Journal of Consulting and Clinical Psychology, 61*(2), 194–198. https://doi.org/10.1037//0022-006x.61.2.194

Beck, J. S. (2011). *Cognitive behavior therapy: Basics and beyond.* New York, NY: Guilford Press.

Biglan, A., Hayes, S. C., & Pistorello, J. (2008). Acceptance and commitment: Implications for prevention science. *Prevention Science, 9*(3), 139–152. https://doi.org/10.1007/s11121-008-0099-4

Brooks, J., Wilson, K., & Amir, Z. (2011). Additional financial costs borne by cancer patients: A narrative review. *European Journal of Oncology Nursing, 15*(4), 302–310. https://doi.org/10.1016/j.ejon.2010.10.005

Burgess, C., Cornelius, V., Love, S., Graham, J., Richards, M., & Ramirez, A. (2005). Depression and anxiety in women with early breast cancer: Five year observational cohort study. *BMJ [British Medical Journal], 330*(7493), 702–705. https://doi.org/10.1136/bmj.38343.670868.D3

Ciaramella, A., & Poli, P. (2001). Assessment of depression among cancer patients: The role of pain, cancer type and treatment. *Psycho-Oncology: Journal of the Psychological, Social and Behavioral Dimensions of Cancer, 10*(2), 156–165. https://doi.org/10.1002/pon.505

Constantinou, M., & Karekla, M. (2015). Experimental design and analysis of single case designs in social sciences. In C. Phellas & D. Valourdos (Eds.), *Research with modern quantitative and qualitative methods in social sciences.* Athens: Papazisis Publications. ISBN: 978-960-2-311-6.

Denham, S. A., Mitchell-Copeland, J., Strandberg, K., Auerbach, S., & Blair, K. (1997). Parental contributions to preschoolers' emotional competence: Direct and indirect effects. *Motivation and Emotion, 21*(1), 65–86. https://doi.org/10.1023/A:1024426431247

Deshields, T., Tibbs, T., Fan, M. Y., & Taylor, M. (2006). Differences in patterns of depression after treatment for breast cancer. *Psycho-Oncology: Journal of the Psychological, Social and Behavioral Dimensions of Cancer, 15*(5), 398–406. https://doi.org/10.1002/pon.962

Fashler, S. R., Weinrib, A. Z., Azam, M. A., & Katz, J. (2018). The use of acceptance and commitment therapy in oncology settings: A narrative review. *Psychological Reports, 121*(2), 229–252. https://doi.org/10.1177/2F0033294117726061

Feldman, G., Hayes, A., Kumar, S., Greeson, J., & Laurenceau, J. P. (2007). Mindfulness and emotion regulation: The development and initial validation of the Cognitive and Affective Mindfulness Scale-Revised (CAMS-R). *Journal of Psychopathology and Behavioral Assessment, 29*(3), 177–190. https://doi.org/10.1007/s10862-006-9035-8

Firsching, V. J., Villanueva, J., Rinner, T. B., Benoy, C., Kuhweide, V., Brogli, S., & Gloster, A. T. (2018). Measuring psychological flexibility in a context sensitive manner - Development and preliminary psychometric properties of a short and accessible questionnaire. In *Poster-Vorstellung anlässlich der ACBS World Conference 16, Montreal, Canada.*

Forman, E. M., Herbert, J. D., Moitra, E., Yeomans, P. D., & Geller, P. A. (2007). A randomized controlled effectiveness trial of acceptance and commitment therapy and cognitive therapy for anxiety and depression. *Behavior Modification, 31*(6), 772–799. https://doi.org/10.1177/2F0145445507302202

Garber, J., Braafladt, N., & Zeman, J. (1991). The regulation of sad affect: An information-processing perspective. In J. Garber & K. A. Dodge (Eds.), *Cambridge studies in social and emotional development. The development of emotion regulation and dysregulation* (pp. 208–240). New York, NY: Cambridge University Press.

Gillanders, D. T., Bolderston, H., Bond, F. W., Dempster, M., Flaxman, P. E., Campbell, L., ... Masley, S. (2014). The development and initial validation of the cognitive fusion questionnaire. *Behavior Therapy, 45*(1), 83–101. https://doi.org/10.1016/j.beth.2013.09.001

Gillanders, D. T., Sinclair, A. K., MacLean, M., & Jardine, K. (2015). Illness cognitions, cognitive fusion, avoidance and self-compassion as predictors of distress and quality of life in a heterogeneous sample of adults, after cancer. *Journal of Contextual Behavioral Science, 4*(4), 300–311. https://doi.org/10.1016/j.jcbs.2015.07.003

Gloster, A. T., Sonntag, R., Hoyer, J., Meyer, A. H., Heinze, S., Ströhle, A., ... Wittchen, H. U. (2015). Treating treatment-resistant patients with panic disorder and agoraphobia using psychotherapy: A randomized controlled switching trial. *Psychotherapy and Psychosomatics, 84*(2), 100–109. https://doi.org/10.1159/000370162

Gregg, J. A. (2013). Self-acceptance and chronic illness. In M. E. Bernard (Ed.), *The strength of self-acceptance* (pp. 247–262). New York, NY: Springer. https://doi. org/10.1007/978-1-4614-6806-6_14

Hack, T. F., & Degner, L. F. (2004). Coping responses following breast cancer diagnosis predict psychological adjustment three years later. *Psycho-Oncology: Journal of the Psychological, Social and Behavioral Dimensions of Cancer, 13*(4), 235–247. https://doi.org/10.1002/pon.739

Hayes, S. C., Barnes-Holmes, D., & Wilson, K. G. (2012). Contextual behavioral science: Creating a science more adequate to the challenge of the human condition. *Journal of Contextual Behavioral Science, 1*(1–2), 1–16. https://doi.org/10.1016/j.jcbs.2012.09.004

Hayes, S. C., & Lillis, J. (2012). *Acceptance and commitment therapy*. Washington, DC: American Psychological Association.

Hayes, S. C., Luoma, J. B., Bond, F. W., Masuda, A., & Lillis, J. (2006). Acceptance and commitment therapy: Model, processes and outcomes. *Behaviour Research and Therapy, 44*(1), 1–25. https://doi.org/10.1016/j.brat.2005.06.006

Hayes, S. C., & Smith, S. (2005). *Get out of your mind and into your life*. Oakland, CA: New Harbinger Publications.

Hayes, S. C., Strosahl, K. D., & Wilson, K. G. (1999). *Acceptance and commitment therapy: An experiential approach to behavior change*. New York, NY: Guilford Press.

Hayes, S. C., Strosahl, K. D., & Wilson, K. G. (2012). *Acceptance and commitment therapy: The process and practice of mindful change* (2nd ed.). New York, NY: Guilford Press.

Hayes, S. C., Wilson, K. G., Gifford, E. V., Follette, V. M., & Strosahl, K. (1996). Experiential avoidance and behavioral disorders: A functional dimensional approach to diagnosis and treatment. *Journal of Consulting and Clinical Psychology, 64*(6), 1152–1168. https://doi.org/1 0.1037/0022-006X.64.6.1152

Hooper, N., Dack, C., Karekla, M., Niyazi, A., & McHugh, L. (2018). Cognitive defusion versus experiential avoidance in the reduction of smoking behaviour: An experimental and preliminary investigation. *Addiction Research and Theory, 26*(5), 414–420. https://doi.org/10.108 0/16066359.2018.1434156

Hopko, D. R., McIndoo, C. C., Gawrysiak, M., & Grassetti, S. (2014). Psychosocial interventions for depressed breast cancer patients. In C. S. Richards & M. W. O'Hara (Eds.), *The oxford handbook of depression and comorbidity* (pp. 546–583). New York, NY: Oxford University Press.

Hulbert-Williams, N. J., Storey, L., & Wilson, K. G. (2015). Psychological interventions for patients with cancer: Psychological flexibility and the potential utility of Acceptance and Commitment Therapy. *European Journal of Cancer Care, 24*(1), 15–27. https://doi.org/10.1111/ecc.12223

Jensen, C. G., Elsass, P., Neustrup, L., Bihal, T., Flyger, H., Kay, S. M., … Würtzen, H. (2014). What to listen for in the consultation. Breast cancer patients' own focus on talking about acceptance-based psychological coping predicts decreased psychological distress and depression. *Patient Education and Counseling, 97*(2), 165–172. https://doi.org/10.1016/j. pec.2014.07.020

Karekla, M., & Constantinou, M. (2010). Religious coping and cancer: Proposing an acceptance and commitment therapy approach. *Cognitive and Behavioral Practice, 17*(4), 371–381. https://doi.org/10.1016/j.cbpra.2009.08.003

Karekla, M., Georgiou, N., Panayiotou, G. P., Sandoz, E., Kurz, S., & Constantinou, M. (2020). Cognitive restructuring vs. defusion: Impact on craving, healthy and unhealthy food intake. *Eating Behaviors, 37*, 101385. https://doi.org/10.1016/j.eatbeh.2020.101385

Karekla, M., Karademas, E., & Gloster, A. (2019). The common sense model of self-regulation and acceptance and commitment therapy: Integrating strategies to guide interventions for chronic illness. *Health Psychology Review, 13*, 490–503. https://doi.org/10.1080/1743719 9.2018.1437550

Karekla, M., Konstantinou, P., Ioannou, M., Kareklas, I., & Gloster, A. T. (2019). The phenomenon of treatment dropout, reasons and moderators in Acceptance and Commitment Therapy and other active treatments: A meta-analytic review. *Clinical Psychology in Europe, 1*(3), e33058. https://doi.org/10.32872/cpe.v1i3.33058

Karekla, M., & Michaelides, M. P. (2017). Validation and invariance testing of the Greek adaptation of the Acceptance and Action Questionnaire-II across clinical vs. nonclinical samples and sexes. *Journal of Contextual Behavioral Science, 6*(1), 119–124. https://doi.org/10.1016/j.jcbs.2016.11.006

Karekla, M., Zacharia, M., & Koushiou, M. (2018). Accept pain for a vital life: Acceptance and commitment therapy for the treatment of chronic pain. In C. Charis & G. Panayiotou (Eds.), *A dialogue between contemporary psychodynamic psychotherapy and cognitive behavioral therapy perspectives* (pp. 163–191). Cham: Springer International Publishing AG. https://doi.org/10.1007/978-3-319-89360-0_10

Kashdan, T. B., & Rottenberg, J. (2010). Psychological flexibility as a fundamental aspect of health. *Clinical Psychology Review, 30*(7), 865–878. https://doi.org/10.1016/j.cpr.2010.03.001

Kissane, D. W., Maj, M., & Sartorius, N. (2011). *Depression and cancer.* Oxford: John Wiley and Sons.

Kyllönen, H. M., Muotka, J., Puolakanaho, A., Astikainen, P., Keinonen, K., & Lappalainen, R. (2018). A brief acceptance and commitment therapy intervention for depression: A randomized controlled trial with 3-year follow-up for the intervention group. *Journal of Contextual Behavioral Science, 10,* 55–63. https://doi.org/10.1016/j.jcbs.2018.08.009

Laurila, J. V., Laakkonen, M. L., Laurila, J. V., Timo, S. E., & Reijo, T. S. (2008). Predisposing and precipitating factors for delirium in a frail geriatric population. *Journal of Psychosomatic Research, 65*(3), 249–254. https://doi.org/10.1016/j.jpsychores.2008.05.026

Lueboonthavatchai, P. (2007). Prevalence and psychosocial factors of anxiety and depression in breast cancer patients. *Journal of the Medical Association of Thailand, 90*(10), 2164–2174. Retrieved from https://pdfs.semanticscholar.org/6a77/3caace82c5195b4f021067dfce41c004a601.pdf

Luoma, J., & Hayes, S. C. (2003). Cognitive defusion. In W. T. Donohue, J. E. Fisher, & S. C. Hayes (Eds.), *Empirically supported techniques for cognitive behavior therapy: A step by step guide for clinicians* (pp. 71–78). New York, NY: Wiley.

Luoma, J. B., Hayes, S. C., & Walser, R. D. (2007). *Learning ACT: An acceptance & commitment therapy skills-training manual for therapists.* Oakland, CA: New Harbinger Publications, Inc..

Luoma, J. B., Hayes, S. C., & Walser, R. D. (2017). *Learning ACT: An acceptance & commitment therapy skills-training manual for therapists* (2nd ed.). Oakland, CA: New Harbinger Publications, Inc..

McCaul, K. D., Sandgren, A. K., King, B., O'Donnell, S., Branstetter, A., & Foreman, G. (1999). Coping and adjustment to breast cancer. *Psycho-Oncology: Journal of the Psychological, Social and Behavioral Dimensions of Cancer, 8*(3), 230–236. https://doi.org/10.1002/(SICI)1099-1611(199905/06)8:3%3C230::AID-PON374%3E3.0.CO;2-%23

McLaughlin, K. A., Conron, K. J., Koenen, K. C., & Gilman, S. E. (2010). Childhood adversity, adult stressful life events, and risk of past-year psychiatric disorder: A test of the stress sensitization hypothesis in a population-based sample of adults. *Psychological Medicine, 40*(10), 1647–1658. https://doi.org/10.1017/S0033291709992121

Monestès, J. L., Karekla, M., Jacobs, N., Michaelides, M., Hooper, N., Kleen, M., … Hayes, S. C. (2018). Experiential avoidance as a common process in European Cultures. *European Journal of Psychological Assessment, 34*(4), 247–257. https://doi.org/10.1027/1015-5759/a000327

Morris, A. S., Silk, J. S., Steinberg, L., Myers, S. S., & Robinson, L. R. (2007). The role of the family context in the development of emotion regulation. *Social Development, 16*(2), 361–388. https://doi.org/10.1111/j.1467-9507.2007.00389.x

Nabors, L. (2020). Depression and anxiety in children. In *Anxiety management in children with mental and physical health problems* (pp. 37–52). Cham: Springer. https://doi.org/10.1007/978-3-030-35606-4_3

Najvani, B. D., Neshatdoost, H. T., Abedi, M. R., & Mokarian, F. (2015). The effect of acceptance and commitment therapy on depression and psychological flexibility in women with breast cancer. *Zahedan Journal of Research in Medical Sciences, 17*(4), 29–33. https://doi.org/10.17795/zjrms965

Nolen-Hoeksema, S. (1991). Responses to depression and their effects on the duration of depressive episodes. *Journal of Abnormal Psychology, 100*(4), 569–582. https://doi.org/10.1037//0021-843x.100.4.569

Páez, M., Luciano, M. C., & Gutiérrez, O. (2007). Psychological treatment for breast cancer: Comparison between acceptance based and cognitive control based strategies. *Psycooncologia, 4*, 75–95.

Paraskeva-Siamata, M., Spyridou, G., Gloster, A., & Karekla, M., (2018, July). *Psyflex: Validation of a new psychological flexibility measure in a Greek-Cypriot sample.* Poster presented at the Association of Contextual Behavior Science annual world conference, Montreal, Canada.

Persons, J. B. (2008). *The case formulation approach to cognitive-behavior therapy.* New York, NY: Guilford Press.

Politi, M. C., Enright, T. M., & Weihs, K. L. (2007). The effects of age and emotional acceptance on distress among breast cancer patients. *Supportive Care in Cancer, 15*(1), 73–79. https://doi.org/10.1007/s00520-006-0098-6

Purdon, C. (1999). Thought suppression and psychopathology. *Behaviour Research and Therapy, 37*(11), 1029–1054. https://doi.org/10.1016/S0005-7967(98)00200-9

Ramnero, J., & Torneke, N. (2008). *The ABCs of human behavior: An introduction to behavioral psychology.* Oakland, CA: New Harbinger Publications, Inc..

Roesch, S. C., Adams, L., Hines, A., Palmores, A., Vyas, P., Tran, C., … Vaughn, A. A. (2005). Coping with prostate cancer: A meta-analytic review. *Journal of Behavioral Medicine, 28*(3), 281–293. https://doi.org/10.1007/s10865-005-4664-z

Rost, A. D., Wilson, K., Buchanan, E., Hildebrandt, M. J., & Mutch, D. (2012). Improving psychological adjustment among late-stage ovarian cancer patients: Examining the role of avoidance in treatment. *Cognitive and Behavioral Practice, 19*(4), 508–517. https://doi.org/10.1016/j.cbpra.2012.01.003

Schotte, C. K. W., Van Den Bossche, B., De Doncker, D., Claes, S., & Cosyns, P. (2006). A biopsychosocial model as a guide for psychoeducation and treatment of depression. *Depression and Anxiety, 23*, 312–324. https://doi.org/10.1002/da.20177

Silk, J. S., Shaw, D. S., Prout, J. T., O'Rourke, F., Lane, T. J., & Kovacs, M. (2011). Socialization of emotion and offspring internalizing symptoms in mothers with childhood-onset depression. *Journal of Applied Developmental Psychology, 32*(3), 127–136. https://doi.org/10.1016/j.appdev.2011.02.001

Silk, J. S., Shaw, D. S., Skuban, E. M., Oland, A. A., & Kovacs, M. (2006). Emotion regulation strategies in offspring of childhood-onset depressed mothers. *Journal of Child Psychology and Psychiatry, 47*(1), 69–78. https://doi.org/10.1111/j.1469-7610.2005.01440.x

Stanton, A. L., Danoff-burg, S., & Huggins, M. E. (2002). The first year after breast cancer diagnosis: Hope and coping strategies as predictors of adjustment. *Psycho-Oncology: Journal of the Psychological, Social and Behavioral Dimensions of Cancer, 11*(2), 93–102. https://doi.org/10.1002/pon.574

Theofanous, A., Ioannou, M., Zacharia, M., Georgiou, S. N., & Karekla, M. (2020). Gender, age, and time invariance of the child and adolescent mindfulness measure (CAMM) and psychometric properties in three Greek-speaking youth samples. *Mindfulness, 11*, 1298. https://doi.org/10.1007/s12671-020-01350-5

Twohig, M. P., & Levin, M. E. (2017). Acceptance and commitment therapy as a treatment for anxiety and depression: A review. *Psychiatric Clinics, 40*(4), 751–770.

Vasiliou, V. S., Michaelides, M. P., Kasinopoulos, O., & Karekla, M. (2019). Psychological Inflexibility in Pain Scale: Greek adaptation, psychometric properties, and invariance testing across three pain samples. *Psychological Assessment, 31*(7), 895904. https://doi.org/10.1037/pas0000705

Veehof, M. M., Trompetter, H. R., Bohlmeijer, E. T., & Schreurs, K. M. G. (2016). Acceptance- and mindfulness-based interventions for the treatment of chronic pain: A meta-analytic review. *Cognitive Behaviour Therapy, 45*(1), 5–31. https://doi.org/10.1080/16506073.2015.1098724

Wetherell, J. L., Afari, N., Rutledge, T., Sorrell, J. T., Stoddard, J. A., Petkus, A. J., … Atkinson, J. H. (2011). A randomized, controlled trial of acceptance and commitment therapy and cognitive-behavioral therapy for chronic pain. *Pain, 152*(9), 2098–2107. https://doi. org/10.1016/j.pain.2011.05.016

Wetter, E. K., & Hankin, B. L. (2009). Mediational pathways through which positive and negative emotionality contribute to anhedonic symptoms of depression: A prospective study of adolescents. *Journal of Abnormal Child Psychology, 37*(4), 507–520. https://doi.org/10.1007/s10802-009-9299-z

Wilkinson, S., & Kitzinger, C. (2000). Thinking differently about thinking positive: A discursive approach to cancer patients' talk. *Social Science & Medicine, 50*(6), 797–811. https://doi. org/10.1016/S0277-9536(99)00337-8

Wilson, K. G. (2009). *Mindfulness for two: An acceptance and commitment therapy approach to mindfulness in psychotherapy*. Oakland, CA: New Harbinger Publications.

Wilson, K. G., & Dufrene, T. (2009). *Mindfulness for two: An acceptance and commitment therapy approach to mindfulness in psychotherapy*. Oakland, CA: New Harbinger.

Wilson, K. G., & Sandoz, E. K. (2008). Mindfulness, values, and the therapeutic relationship in acceptance and commitment therapy. In S. Hick & T. Bein (Eds.), *Mindfulness and the therapeutic relationship* (pp. 89–106). New York, NY: Guilford Press.

Wilson, K. G., Sandoz, E. K., Kitchens, J., & Roberts, M. (2010). The valued living questionnaire: Defining and measuring valued action within a behavioral framework. *The Psychological Record, 60*(2), 249–272. https://doi.org/10.1007/BF03395706

Wilson, S., DiRago, A. C., & Iacono, W. G. (2014). Prospective inter-relationships between late adolescent personality and major depressive disorder in early adulthood. *Psychological Medicine, 44*(3), 567–577. https://doi.org/10.1017/S0033291713001104

Yan, R., Xia, J., Yang, R., Lv, B., Wu, P., Chen, W., … Yu, J. (2019). Association between anxiety, depression, and comorbid chronic diseases among cancer survivors. *Psycho-Oncology, 28*(6), 1269–1277. https://doi.org/10.1002/pon.5078

Yap, M. B., Allen, N. B., & Ladouceur, C. D. (2008). Maternal socialization of positive affect: The impact of invalidation on adolescent emotion regulation and depressive symptomatology. *Child Development, 79*(5), 1415–1431. https://doi.org/10.1111/j.1467-8624.2008.01196.x

Zabora, J., BrintzenhofeSzoc, K., Curbow, B., Hooker, C., & Piantadosi, S. (2001). The prevalence of psychological distress by cancer site. *Psycho-Oncology: Journal of the Psychological, Social and Behavioral Dimensions of Cancer, 10*(1), 19–28. https://doi.org/10.1002/1099-161 1(200101/02)10:1%3C19::AID-PON501%3E3.0.CO;2-6

Zacharia, M., Ioannou, M., Theofanous, A., Vasiliou, V. S., & Karekla, M. (2021). Does Cognitive Fusion show up similarly across two behavioral health samples? Psychometric properties and invariance of the Greek–Cognitive Fusion Questionnaire (G-CFQ). *Journal of Contextual Behavioral Science*. https://doi.org/10.1016/j.jcbs.2021.01.003

Zafar, S. Y., Alexander, S. C., Weinfurt, K. P., Schulman, K. A., & Abernethy, A. P. (2009). Decision making and quality of life in the treatment of cancer: A review. *Supportive Care in Cancer, 17*(2), 117–127. https://doi.org/10.1007/s00520-008-0505-2

Zettle, R. (2007). *ACT for depression: A clinician's guide to using acceptance & commitment therapy in treating depression*. Oakland, CA: New Harbinger.

Zhang, C. Q., Leeming, E., Smith, P., Chung, P. K., Hagger, M. S., & Hayes, S. C. (2018). Acceptance and commitment therapy for health behavior change: A contextually-driven approach. *Frontiers in Psychology, 8*, 2350.

Zigmond, A. S., & Snaith, R. P. (1983). The hospital anxiety and depression scale. *Acta Psychiatrica Scandinavica, 67*(6), 361–370. https://doi.org/10.1111/j.1600-0447.1983. tb09716.x

Chapter 10
Application of a Manualized Cognitive-Behavioral Treatment Protocol to an Individual with Bipolar Disorder in a Private Practice Setting

Eleni Karayianni

Contents

CBT is widely used for depression and there is plenty of evidence to support its efficacy. However, its support for treating bipolar disorder is still modest, and where it is strongly supported as a form of treatment, it mostly refers to mania or depression separately. Even though pharmacological treatment remains broadly the go-to intervention modality for treating bipolar patients, research on its efficacy has produced mixed results (Geddes & Miklowitz, 2013). Thus, focusing only on addressing the biological aspects of bipolar disorder has several limitations. Geddes and Miklowitz (2013) supported that to achieve best results in treating bipolar disorder, professionals and researchers ought to continue to strive for combination in addressing the neurobiological and psychosocial underpinnings, as well as modifying treatments to suit the needs of the individuals diagnosed with the disorder.

E. Karayianni (✉)
University of Cyprus, Nicosia, Cyprus
e-mail: ekarayia@ucy.ac.cy

© Springer Nature Switzerland AG 2021
C. Charis, G. Panayiotou (eds.), *Depression Conceptualization and Treatment*,
https://doi.org/10.1007/978-3-030-68932-2_10

Swartz and Swanson (2014), in their systematic review of bipolar-focused treatments, reported that combining psychotherapies targeting bipolar disorder specifically to medication treatment proved to be superior every time to medication alone, especially in reducing symptoms and improving relapse prevention. A more recent meta-analysis by Chiang et al. (2017) focused more on the efficacy of CBT as a psychotherapeutic mode of treatment for bipolar disorder. The authors noted the need to explore the efficacy of CBT for bipolar disorder since it had shown to be promising as an adjunct to pharmacotherapy. Results from reviewing 19 RCTs with 1384 bipolar I or II patients supported that CBT had mild to moderate effect sizes in reducing relapse rates, improving depressive symptoms, mania severity, and overall psychosocial functioning.

10.1 Case Introduction

The case report will describe the background, treatment, and outcome of the application of a manualized cognitive-behavioral therapy protocol in a private practice setting. To protect the client's confidentiality, the pseudonym "Anna" will be used in the discussion of the case. Demographic and other information have also been altered to further protect identification of the client. The author is grateful to the client, who provided permission to use their clinical information for the purpose of the case presentation.

At the time of the referral, Anna was a married woman in her late 30s who sought treatment following an episode of major depression. She was recommended to therapy by her then psychiatrist who indicated that she needed to "build up resilience" and to "identify and cope with stressors."

10.2 Presenting Complaints

Anna reported the onset of depressive symptoms 6 months prior to her coming to therapy. The onset appeared to be due to "feeling like a failure" following work-related financial problems and having to close her small family business. Anna reported having reduced appetite, no motivation to work, fatigue and inability to sustain sleep, poor concentration, hopelessness, anhedonia, and feeling unable to emotionally respond to her young child (feeling "soulless"). She indicated that having to close down the business that left her husband without a job, the communication issues with her father who was trying to help her family financially by offering Anna and her husband work in his family business, and her failure to gain pleasure from her new job role were the top three factors causing her distress.

While she had been prescribed SSRIs by the psychiatrist since the beginning of the current episode, she continued to exhibit several symptoms that affected her daily functioning. As a result, she reported feeling "incompetent," that her self-esteem had been impacted negatively, and she took on the blame for all the family failures. With these in mind, the identified goals in seeking psychological services were to clarify her future professional steps, to address her relationship with her father and the communication issues that arise from the tension between them, and to set boundaries between the roles she tries to fulfill in her daily life.

10.3   History

Anna stated that she had experienced one other episode of depression in the past but had never sought systematic treatment before. The episode developed following a return to her home country from studying abroad. She indicated that her family placed great pressure on her to return with her then boyfriend and to marry. In addition, there was the expectation of her joining the family business. She went forward with fulfilling all three expectations in order to appease her father and because she felt she could not do otherwise. At the time, her boyfriend provided her with what she felt was enough support to get through the episode without seeking any medical or psychological assistance. She also reported having a stable source of support from friends throughout her life as she was outgoing and always actively involved in various social activities.

The family of origin was reported to be very close. Anna felt closer to her mother due to her mild-mannered nature and for receiving support in her role as a mother. On the other hand, her relationship with her father was reported to have been conflictual due to father's high and strict expectations. She reported having good relations with her brother and his family. However, she reported that she always felt that her father had higher expectations of her. These expectations put a lot of pressure on her from a young age and apparently this didn't change with time. All family members either were or have worked at the family-owned business. Anna invested a lot of her time to the job and used to find great pleasure in promoting the business. Even though the business was quite successful, it was also a cause of great distress and arguments between the family members. Differences of opinion with regard to handling changes in the business led to greater interpersonal difficulties, which in turn led to her husband leaving the business and her doing the same some years later. Following these major employment changes, business investments left her and her husband exposed to financial instability and threat. She managed to rebuild the business and had to seek additional work via her father's family business once more in order to safeguard her family's finances.

Anna's family has a long history of mental health issues. Her mother reportedly has experienced several depressive episodes throughout the client's lifetime. Moreover, Anna's brother and a cousin had also been diagnosed with depression with psychotic symptoms and had sought medical treatment outside the country. Anna stated that her father was very critical and unaccepting of the diagnosis, while her mother was very supportive despite feeling sadness for both her children having been diagnosed with depression. Her and her family's medical history is unremarkable. She also denied any current use of illegal substances at the time of the initial assessment but did report smoking heavily on a daily basis, due to increased stress, and being a social drinker. She did report a previous history of using cannabis with her husband. However, she stated that she had managed to stop the use on her own some time before the episode onset.

10.4 Assessment Strategies

One of the main challenges in working with Anna was assessing objectively her baseline functioning at the time of referral, as well as assessing treatment effectiveness throughout and at the end of the intervention. While measures have been translated in Greek and are used in research and practice alike, very few of those are standardized in the local population. This makes it particularly difficult to extract any accurate results and to infer conclusions. Of those standardized, very few would have been appropriate for assessing the present case, and they are not widely available for use outside of research centers. Thus, there were ethical and legal obstacles to consider. Therefore, treatment effectiveness was primarily measured by the client's report of increased psychological stability and witnessed by the therapist, as well as reports from family and friends who were identified as being key support people to Anna.

Based on the initial assessment and the consultation with the psychiatrist, the original diagnosis given was major depressive disorder, severe without psychotic features, recurrent. However, as will be discussed below, based on information obtained during treatment and other observations, the diagnosis was changed to bipolar I disorder and cannabis use disorder.

10.5 Clinical Case Formulation

Anna reported having fragile self-esteem as she has always found the approval of others very important. At the time of intake, she felt that she had reached one of her lowest points due to thinking that she had let everyone in her immediate and extended family down as a daughter, a wife, a mother, and an employee. Subsequent to the negative thoughts and evaluation of her experiences, symptoms of depression began. Ongoing conflict between her spouse and her family of origin also contributed to the worsening of her relationship with both her husband and her father. As a result of these intra- and interfamilial problems, the depressive symptomatology worsened. Thus, a connection has evolved between her depressive symptoms, the interpersonal problems experienced within the family and work settings that are interconnected, and her negative cognitions. The levels of dysfunction in her family and the conflict contributing to her relapses are supported by research indicating that expressed emotion in such families can pose a very high risk for the individual as can the occurrence of negative life events (e.g., Johnson & Miller, 1997; Miklowitz et al., 1988). Furthermore, negative cognitive styles have also been found to be interconnected to depressive attitudes and attributional styles when combined with negative life events (e.g., Reilly-Harrington et al., 1999). Both appear to hold true in Anna's case.

At the same time, her manic episodes were also clearly connected to her negative cognitions and in trying to overcompensate for her core beliefs developed as a child that she "has to be good to be loved and respected" or that she is "worthless." In her attempts to prove her loved ones wrong about what she perceived their view of her to be, she would engage in behaviors that were self-destructive (e.g., taking on a lot of responsibility for the family business' success, trying to manage too many things at the same time and be perfect at them). Cycling through the lowered and elevated mood was inevitable, especially as she used cannabis and/or alcohol at times on a consistent basis to regulate the changes.

On the basis of the relationship among her problems, Anna and the therapist decided to address her negative thinking first before tackling the interpersonal difficulties in an attempt to give her time to adjust her view of herself, to develop sufficient coping skills, and to then tackle issues that left her feeling most vulnerable to negative self-criticism. Her symptoms of depression and her cannabis use were not included as goals in the treatment plan. It was assumed, on the basis of the relationship among the various difficulties, that such complaints would also diminish as the thinking and behaviors would become more balanced and as the interpersonal problems would be addressed since these were identified as the major triggers to these problems.

10.6   Treatment

10.6.1   Choice of Treatment

In choosing a treatment model for Anna, her presenting problem of depression led to choosing CBT as the treatment of choice given the body of evidence supporting its effectiveness. Once the diagnosis was changed to bipolar disorder, it only seemed natural to maintain the same treatment modality because the client appeared to respond positively to the structured format of the work. According to Otto, Reilley-Harrington, and Sachs (2003), CBT has been found to benefit progress in treating bipolar disorder. It has been identified that CBT for bipolar disorder targets six areas. These areas concern relapse prevention, medication adherence, early detection and intervention, stress and lifestyle management, treatment of comorbid conditions, and treatment of bipolar depression (Otto et al., 2003).

Otto et al.'s (2009) CBT guide was chosen even though it clearly states that it is targeted for patients receiving treatment in specialist clinics for bipolar disorder. The primary reason for the choice had to do with the fact that Otto et al. developed the program with a focus on relapse prevention particularly in high-risk situations. This seemed to fit Anna's identified needs.

The guide outlines an up to 30-session program separated into 4 sections: the depression phase; the contract phase; the problems-list phase; and the well-being phase. Treatment Phase 1 (Sessions 1–9) concentrates on establishing mood stability by mood charting and activity scheduling, cognitive restructuring, and core beliefs work. Treatment Phase 2 (Sessions 10–13) is the contract phase. Treatment Phase 3 sees the client build skills such as problem-solving, social skills, relaxation, and anger management. Treatment Phase 4, the last one, helps the client pay attention to improving well-being and the end of treatment. The program also has a family component wherein the client's family members attend psychoeducation sessions to learn more about the disorder and they have to work with the client and the therapist to achieve best results (Otto et al., 2009).

10.6.2   Treatment Implementation

Overall, treatment lasted 1.5 years in total including the follow-up sessions and amounted to 44 sessions in total, covering materials at a varying rate depending on Anna's progress and life events. All sessions lasted 45–60 min. The case study focuses on how CBT for bipolar disorder was used with Anna and in particular how it was delivered in the context of a private practice taking into consideration risk and additional complexity. The manual was used throughout treatment, and the exercises assigned for homework or completed during session were the ones outlined within the manual.

10.6.3   Treatment Phase 1

Sessions 1 and 2   Engagement and Rationale for Treatment: In the first two sessions, Anna provided extensive background information relating to her current and past difficulties, the most recent depressive episode, intrafamilial problems, and other psychosocial issues that contributed to her experiencing mental health difficulties. Session 1 focused on history taking of interpersonal and financial issues, and assessing current functioning.

Session 2, on the other hand, focused on Anna identifying her primary goals, as well as identifying her own strengths and weaknesses. As noted above, Anna's main goals were to define what she will do with her professional life, how to set clear boundaries in her different roles, and how to improve communication with her father by being more assertive and less fearful of his reactions to her choices. In terms of weaknesses, she identified that she can be very stubborn especially when she is wrong and that she holds grudges. Perhaps her biggest negative attribute was her engaging in significant self-blaming when something felt like a failure or went wrong, by taking on more responsibility than was due. Her dynamic personality was identified as both a positive and negative attribute that contributed to her perseverance all these years but also gave her trouble when she needed to be focused on tasks. Anna identified that she was kind, full of love for her family and friends, giving and supportive to her loved ones, and an all-around pleasant person to be in the company of. Contact with her first psychiatrist was done as part of the assessment phase in order to coordinate treatment and establish shared therapeutic goals. Furthermore, the rationale of the model used was emphasized.

Sessions 3–7 Cognitive Restructuring: Cognitive restructuring was introduced in Session 3, as is in the manual, without covering mood charting and activity scheduling first. The rationale was that the client reported experiencing increased distress over "negative thinking." The session was primarily spent on psychoeducation around automatic thoughts, the distortions, and the purpose of completing thought records. This led to her admitting in the following session that she "wants to feel loved by everyone!" The statement was examined in the context of her life's meaning and motivation for her actions but also as a source of distress, disappointment, and unrealistic expectations. Homework continued to be in the form of completing thought records.

Session 5 was spent identifying scenarios throughout the week relating to the aforementioned statement and to her depression in general as she did not complete the written component of the homework. Anna easily identified events and automatic thoughts and was able to work through the thought records in session identifying where her thinking was unrealistic and where it set a precedent for feeling depressed. The main themes identified related to interpersonal difficulties at home. Mood charting and activity scheduling were also introduced to monitor symptoms and activity levels.

Session 6 was planned for continued work on cognitive restructuring, mood charting, and activity scheduling. However, several instances of conflict in the family during the previous week steered Anna into experiencing mood swings and impulses for reducing medication and several "good ideas" for businesses, reduced sleep, and other difficulties. Contact with the psychiatrist proved difficult, and a recommendation for finding a local-based doctor was made. A short behavioral management plan was created where Anna had to follow two rules before acting on her impulsive thinking: (a) a "48 h Before Acting Rule" where clients are encouraged to wait at least 2 full days with 2 full nights' sleep before acting on new ideas or plans and (b) a "Two-Person Feedback Rule" where at least two trusted people have to help the client to test whether an idea or plan is good (Newman, Leahy, Beck, Reilly-Harrington, & Gyulai, 2001). It was also agreed that no major decisions or life changes would be made during a manic or depressive episode. Anna agreed with the plan and decided that she wished for the one person of the two to be the therapist. The family was asked to attend the next session. Thus, the following session was attended by Anna with her husband and mother. There was a medication change and Seroquel was added to the standard SSRI. The family was provided with psychoeducation on bipolar disorder.

Sessions 8–12 Redefining Treatment and Establishing Support: A full-on manic episode was reported by Session 8 by Anna's husband as she had not been taking her medication as prescribed. Anna reported that her negative thoughts and feeling "unappreciated" reached a level where she thought that stopping would help her be more productive. She counterbalanced her elevated mood by smoking cannabis daily. Furthermore, Anna reported that she had previously had experiences of elevated mood where she also exhibited increased religiosity, once to the point of feeling like she had special healing powers. She negated having similar experiences since that one time but was concerned about it and felt ashamed. A change to a local psychiatrist was made in order to better monitor medication intake. We reviewed treatment goals and provided psychoeducation on mania and its management. By Session 9, Anna had achieved some mood stability, and we resumed treatment by focusing on cognitive distortions around mania and hypomania. Coping skills (e.g., progressive muscle relaxation) were also reviewed, and the need to have regular activity planning (e.g., exercise) was revisited.

Session 10 continued to cover activity scheduling and introduced weekly planning to help Anna achieve a balance in number of activities, their intensity, and time investment as it became evident from the thought records that this was a major challenge and destabilizing factor. Unfortunately, Session 11 was cancelled due to having a minor depressive episode and not having completed any of her homework. Anna came to her next session with her husband, who began by doubting the effectiveness of treatment, feeling uncertain about the future, and trusting that either medical or psychological treatment will be effective in helping Anna "get back to her normal self." This was addressed in session with Anna present, who stated her investment to working things through in therapy. Then, the session was redirected to identifying antecedents of the depressive episode and working through thought records to address the mood changes. Given all the intrafamilial difficulties that came to rise and the influence that people's opinion had on Anna and her investment in treatment, it was agreed that the work on core beliefs would be put on hold until the contract phase is completed. Both Anna and the therapist felt that this would minimize therapy-interfering behaviors, as well as help Anna feel more in control of her treatment, her decisions, and her life overall.

10.6.4   Treatment Phase 2

Sessions 13–16 Contract Phase: While the work with the thought records and activity planning was ongoing, work on the second phase of treatment began as Anna's mood became more stable and we wished to start on relapse prevention in Phase 3 following the work on core beliefs.

In Session 13, we reviewed the various mood episodes in order to help Anna start completing her treatment contract. The psychiatrist was also informed of the contract development process. Anna identified the people she'd wish to have as her support system that, apart from the therapist and psychiatrist, included her husband, her mother, and two very close friends. Psychoeducation provided on decision-making skills aimed at helping Anna with her experiencing problems that needed to be addressed within her marriage. The next two sessions continued to review activity scheduling as an ongoing process and to filling in the contract.

In working on the contract in Sessions 14 and 15, Anna was better able to identify the things she does when she is feeling well (e.g., taking care of her appearance on a regular basis, attending work, and keeping up with family and social activities throughout the week) and the things she can do to better help herself feel well (e.g., takes her medication as prescribed, keeps a regular sleep schedule, takes care of family finances). She was able to name her behaviors, thoughts, and emotions that were early signs of depression (e.g., difficulty concentrating, thoughts that others don't care when they really might, having no energy and feeling emotionally numb, having trouble sleeping or sleeping too much, staying away from people, and stopping activities), the triggers (e.g., relationship breakups and especially conflict in the spousal relationship, using drugs or alcohol, difficulties at work), the coping skills needed to effectively address these in terms of things she can do to help herself (e.g., contacting her treatment providers, contacting two specific friends for support, maintaining a regular activity schedule and not staying in bed all day, ensuring that she's taking her medication and is not using substances), and how others can best assist her (e.g., by not doubting her when she's telling them that she is feeling depressed and by contacting her treatment providers). Similarly, Anna identified thoughts, behaviors, and emotions as early signs of elevated mood (e.g., racing thoughts and feeling particularly creative, thoughts of having special powers, feeling inpatient and irritable, doubting that anything bad might happen, excessive talk and being sociable, easily fighting without reason), triggers for hypomania or mania (e.g., relationship breakup, seasonal changes, work-related problems, drug use), and coping skills for herself (e.g., maintaining regular schedule and avoiding substances, contacting support persons), as well as instructions for others (e.g., talk to her trusted people in her support system, talk to the priest who is her spiritual guide, preventing her from driving and putting her in a room with minimal stimulation).

The contract meeting with the support system was planned for Session 16 but instead occurred in Session 17. Anna called previously to the session to report "bad thoughts" about her family, finances, and her relationship, thus needing to take one more session to process these through the thought records. Once that was done, Session 17 was attended by the four people named in her contract as her support system. All attendees, including Anna, found the session and the document as representative of Anna's situation, and a helpful document to follow to best help Anna through her treatment and onward. Anna reported feeling content and proud of herself for the first time in treatment and that she felt in charge of her life.

10.6.5   Treatment Phase 3

Sessions 18–22 Mood Charting and Skills Building: Session 18 started with Anna reporting feeling somewhat elevated mood due to being upset with her husband and their relationship overall. This was an opportunity to introduce problem-solving skills. The work continued into Session 19, where Anna reported reduced mood due to her father calling the therapist for the first time and attempting to influence the treatment process and progress. Anna's concerns regarding their relationship, especially with regard to dysfunctional communication, were addressed in session.

Session 20 addressed anger management skills following another episode where Anna experienced increased agitation and anger toward her husband. The therapist chose to revisit thought records and mood charting with Anna as a means of monitoring her effectiveness and reducing risk of relapse. However, Session 21 revealed that Anna hadn't completed her homework and felt that it ought to be considered necessary only in "serious situations." The therapist provided psychoeducation on the necessity for consistency in order to achieve desirable results in treatment. We went on to discuss interpersonal effectiveness skills, especially in dealing with setting boundaries. Despite her reaction in Session 21, Anna came to Session 22 with her homework done and reporting that it had been "useful" in reviewing her medication with her psychiatrist, in further identifying situations in her daily life that could pose a risk for her, and in putting the use of the contract in place.

Sessions 23–30 Core Beliefs and Skills Building: The first half of the next session focused on reviewing Anna's mood chart. That resulted in spotting dysfunctional behaviors such as increased sleep and increased activity levels in order to catch up for lost time leading to increased irritability and increased mood as a result. While thought records were partially helpful, Anna's ongoing relationship problems with her husband needed to be addressed at a different level. Thus, the therapist referred them to couples' therapy. The second half of the session addressed Anna's concern regarding new job opportunities and the introduction of core beliefs as actively job seeking left Anna troubled as to how to inform her family that she'd be leaving the family business again.

Session 24 dealt with a crisis that related to Anna's relationship with her husband. Both her mother and husband had called the therapist prior to the session in great concern over Anna's mood swings. In session, Anna indicated that she was sensing increased irritability and reactivity with regard to her continuing marital problems and had had mild suicidal ideation, which resulted in her using substances to calm herself down. Contact with the psychiatrist was made to monitor medication intake and to have a session urgently, as well as to assess potential need for hospitalization. Case management via out-of-session contact, implementing the contract with the support system, and having a crisis session with the psychiatrist helped manage the episode without hospitalization.

In Session 25, Anna felt more hopeful primarily because she had another job interview. The therapist worked with Anna on the potential risks for relapse relating to the notable mood swings noted in the last few weeks. Anna stated that while she was "feeling down" because of her relationship with her husband, she felt glad that things were looking up professionally. Anna and the therapist re-addressed challenging core beliefs relating to respect ("I have to be good to be appreciated") and focused on applying her decision-making skills. The same theme continued into Session 26; however Anna reported that because of her keeping up with her medication and sleep schedule, and in reaching out to her support system, she had managed to return to her baseline faster and more effectively. She also stated that couples' work would start the same week. This helped with furthering work on challenging core beliefs. Specifically, Anna identified early-on experiences where she adopted the view that her self-worth depended heavily on her perceived love and respect received from others. These occasions primarily stemmed from interactions with her father and from witnessing her parents' relationship. In addition, Anna identified core beliefs such as "I am incompetent" and "I have to be perfect to be loved."

Session 27 found Anna feeling irritable following the first couple's session. The therapist addressed problem-solving skills and ongoing use of thought records and mood charting as a means of helping with stabilization. Unfortunately, couples' sessions proved to be a major destabilizing factor for Anna, as she came to Session 28 with no homework completed and wishing to discuss only the emotional turmoil that was causing her instability at the time. By Session 29, Anna returned to implementing her homework and feeling more efficient and effective. Skills for interpersonal effectiveness, problem-solving, and anger management were revisited in session. Moreover, assertiveness skills with regard to family interactions were covered as part of Session 30 as Anna reported increased worry regarding family interactions and reduced communication.

Sessions 31–38 Skills Building and Relapse Prevention: In Session 31, Anna reported on her continuous efforts to implement skills learned and how that helped her feel more effective and competent. A review of treatment progress was made and re-worked on the developmental trajectory of goal attainment leading to termination. Anna reinstated her focus on her life goals of becoming independent from parents and to stop being codependent with her husband. She went on to state that her adjusted expectations coincided with adjusting her core beliefs to "I am worthy." In contrast, the next two sessions presented with challenges since Anna reported that her mood had lowered following the most recent couples' session and increased use of cannabis as a result. These events coincided with her feeling angry and disappointed connected to her feeling "incompetent." Thus, work in session focused on remastering skills needed to achieve her goals relating to her core beliefs. This work continued into Session 34.

By Session 35, Anna started actively working on relapse prevention. She reported having started a new job, feeling excited, and higher levels of energy. We revisited triggers for manic episodes and how she regains balance by following her contract. In Session 36, Anna reviewed a recent event that could have presented a threat to her self-esteem and that she reported having managed effectively. We reviewed how her current behavior connected to her adjusted core beliefs and life goals. Session 37 also focused on relapse prevention and maintenance. We reviewed treatment progress and formed termination plan that would include a group meeting of the support system. Anna and the therapist agreed on a maximum of another six sessions including the group and termination sessions. The need to work toward termination was affirmed in Session 38 where Anna reported continuous improvement since she had established a regular schedule by having a stable job, returning to an active social life and to practicing her favorite sport, as well as spending quality time with her son and family.

10.6.6   Treatment Phase 4

Sessions 39–44   Well-Being and Termination: Session 39 introduced the notion of well-being and connected it to her meaning of life as it had been defined in the early sessions and redefined later on while challenging core beliefs and identifying new life goals. This became more evident when she cancelled Session 40 due to having a family activity with her son.

In Session 41, she reported the end of couples' sessions and a goal for ongoing commitment to working on shared issues. With regard to her individual goals, Anna reported experiencing three stressors and having dealt with two effectively on her own. The third one related to her family sharing personal information regarding her diagnosis without her consent. Anna reviewed her plan of action for addressing this issue with the therapist prior to implementing it. The efficiency and mood stability was evident in Session 42 also. Anna stated that she felt she had achieved a substantial amount in treatment and that she "will keep on working on things that need to be addressed." The group session was held during Session 43 where her mother, husband, and two friends attended the session. They were all able to identify notable changes in Anna including her skills and mood stability. Most notably, her husband attempted to question the continued use of medication to which Anna contradicted him stating that she felt she needed even the low dose to help keep her mood stable and would consult only with her psychiatrist and therapist as needed for medication changes.

Session 44 was the termination session. Anna and the therapist appraised treatment as a whole. We reviewed goals attained and the ones that remain ongoing life goals.

10.7 Complicating Factors

In working with Anna, several challenges were identified early on. Both therapist and client addressed them as they were identified and on an ongoing basis in order to achieve stability and reduce relapse.

Firstly, achieving stability in medical treatment proved to be a challenge. The initial obstacle to having stability was that she had initially sought the professional help of her brother's psychiatrist who only practiced part-time in the country. As this was a major challenge to coordinating care, Anna was encouraged to seek the support of a local psychiatrist. Additionally, the use of cannabis played a role in the client's wish to "return to her old self" by reducing her medication at will and without notice particularly when she felt drowsy and using the cannabis to self-medicate. Anna reported "feeling slowed down" by the medication and that she couldn't think or feel as alert as she was prior to beginning the combination of an SSRI and an antipsychotic drug. She would resort in reducing the dosage of the antipsychotic drug, which in turn would lead to a hypomanic or manic episode, which in turn she'd try to slow down by increasing her cannabis use. In turn, that sometimes led to a depressive episode. The added obstacle in this factor was her husband's feedback and verification of these observations that reinforced her behavior. Through ongoing support, psychoeducation, and communication with her family and psychiatrist, the "team" worked together with Anna to reduce the medication to a level that was acceptable to her and that helped her feel more "awake" while keeping her mood stabilized. In time and by the end of treatment, the cannabis use had significantly decreased to the point that she reported no use at closure. A relapse plan was discussed as part of follow-up.

Secondly, initially Anna relied heavily on outside feedback for evaluating her self-worth. As a result, she suffered from the instability in her relationship with her husband. About a third of the time into treatment, it became apparent that her decision-making relating to her health and life in general was heavily influenced by her husband's feedback on her appearance, her functioning, and her role as a mother and wife. From being her biggest supporter, he ended up being her biggest critic and thus her biggest trigger for either a depressive or manic episode. This contributed greatly to her relapses but also to her returning more determined to work on believing in herself, to focus on restructuring her core beliefs to reflect her view of herself and the world, and to work on maintenance. Similarly, her family's initial reaction to the diagnosis and treatment left the client feeling unloved and rejected. This was especially true of her father's reaction. While her mother came in for the contract meeting and subsequent family meetings, her father refused to come in but continued to "monitor" treatment by calling the therapist. This was addressed in time by the therapist and with coordinated action by Anna. In the end, her family of origin was a stable support system that encouraged her to re-establish herself.

One final factor is that of applying a phasic model of treatment in a "real-world," private practice setting. Several challenges outlined above and below occurred that contributed to derailing the treatment plan following the contract phase. The therapist had to revisit skills with Anna and to work on helping her stabilize her mood and re-establish the indicated route by the manual authors. However, framing these episodes which Anna identified as "failures" as an anticipated part of an ongoing process in life helped reduce the shame and to work through the episodes one at a time, regardless of how difficult they were emotionally, or how slow the process. This also meant that the treatment was individualized to address Anna's needs.

10.8   Follow-Up

Follow-up sessions were completed as indicated by Otto et al. (2009) at 1, 3, and 6 months post-treatment. At these reviews, Anna described what skills she had been practicing well and how she had used her skills to support herself. She reflected on the things that continued to trouble her and the concerns that connect to these troubles. Her primary concern at the time of follow-up was her relationship with her husband and how their ongoing issues would be resolved. She maintained that she was coping well with the ups and downs but that the decision-making process was proving to be especially complicated. Nonetheless, her mood was relatively well balanced primarily due to keeping up with her medication regime, her work schedule, social life, and motherhood. Therefore, while she had achieved her goal of becoming independent from her family of origin, her goal of working on her relationship with her husband remained. Planning for positive events was not an issue any more, and the support she received from those close to her was reported as ongoing. Remarkably, as a "side effect" to treatment, her cannabis use had reduced significantly to the point of not having used since the end of treatment.

10.9   Discussion

This case study illustrates how a structured psychotherapeutic intervention for bipolar disorder can be effective even with several confounding variables. It is recognized that only tentative conclusions can be drawn from a single case study.

10.9.1   Treatment Implications of the Case

One of the major factors that appeared clearly to play a role in the progress and process of therapy in this case was the development of a good, solid therapeutic relationship with the client. While it can be considered a given in any therapeutic model that for therapy to work one needs to establish a good therapeutic relationship to start with, it cannot be emphasized enough when applying a manualized treatment. Beck, Rush, Shaw, and Emery (1979) termed this "collaborative empiricism," where the client and therapist form a team to work together in researching cognitions. Moreover, it has been found that the strength of the treatment alliance can predict fewer manic symptoms (Strauss & Johnson, 2012). In this case, it helped with the client feeling trust in the therapist and the therapist's intention to help the client through life's difficulties, as well as feel accepted without being judged or scrutinized for her "failures" in life. It was evident in the reduced sense of shame experienced by the client whenever there was a relapse in that she was not afraid to be honest in therapy, to report the incident, and to work together with the therapist and her support network to get back on track. This is of importance as shame can be a major destabilizing factor in treatment progress and outcome (McMurrich & Johnson, 2009).

Moreover, the opportunity to build a safety network with the use of the contract offered opportunities to promote growth in the client and concurrently ensure her and her child's safety in crisis situations. By identifying and naming her own triggers and coping skills, and by communicating these to the people she chose to have surround her while in treatment, the client reported feeling in control of her treatment, that people respected her wishes and followed her lead in providing the assistance she felt and identified as being the most helpful for her when she was the most vulnerable and feeling "out of control" with life. In turn, the safety network expressed a sense of relief and competence in knowing what to do, how to do it, and when to do it since they were given clear behavioral benchmarks by which to assess the client's functioning and well-being, rather than assuming action based on their own understanding and assessment of the situation. For them, having access to the therapist assisted in providing another level of security.

In line with the medication effectiveness research, the medication regime proved to be a challenge and a critical aspect in Anna's stabilization. One of the factors that contributed to medication adherence in this case on an individual level was the experience of relapses with significant mood swings and the aftermath of these relapses. The intermittent questioning of the medication, its use and usefulness, as well as what constitutes the necessary or desirable dosage for Anna to feel stable but not blunt led to her seizing her medication at different occasions. The resulting instability, especially when she experienced another depressive episode, was detrimental to her changing her mind, collaborating with her psychiatrist, and sticking to the agreed regime. Moreover, through psychoeducation and ongoing support by the therapist and her support system, the client worked with her psychiatrist to regulate the medication at a level that was effective for her.

One final major challenge was the treatment itself. On one hand, having a treatment team offering services under one roof in a "one stop shop" format has noted benefits when managing cases that require coordinated care. This is especially true when applying a manualized treatment in an individual-based setting. Even though the therapist and psychiatrist were in close and ongoing contact, consistent communication was not feasible between two people working out of two separate private practices due to practical reasons (e.g., being able to reach each other over the phone and depending on availability to talk). On the other hand, one needs to take into consideration the costs of providing such services in a private practice setting.

The up to 30 sessions plan proposed by Otto et al. proved to be unfeasible in this case given the relapses that occurred while Anna was in treatment. The treatment for both psychotherapy and medication was covered out of pocket as mental health services are not a modality that are usually covered in their totality by health insurance plans. In addition, manualized treatments are not oftentimes offered in the public mental health system where clients have access to services at a reduced cost due to variability in psychologists' psychotherapy training. Thus, costs can accrue or be prohibitive for an individual seeking treatment.

10.9.2   Recommendations to Clinicians and Trainees

It is essential to accurately assess the client's situation and context. This will enable the therapist to identify and choose the best modality of treatment for them while placing an emphasis on using evidence-based treatments. This approach will help reduce identified risks, promote collaborative services, and provide structure especially for clients who report "feeling out of control."

At the same time, when considering the application of manualized treatment in a "real-life" setting, one has to take into consideration the obstacles that may arise and the need to have and to give the client the time they need, thus providing an individualized plan of action. In the context of Anna's case, this meant alternating between phases based on what was needed and going over the recommended number of sessions to give both the therapist and the client the time to reflect, recover, and truly focus on the treatment. The added sessions didn't necessarily cover new materials or ones already covered. Rather, they focused on going over with Anna's practical behavioral strategies as a response to dealing with the transient or ongoing at times negative cognitions and distortions. This is based on the concept of "flexibility within fidelity" coined by Kendall and colleagues (Kendall & Frank, 2018; Kendall, Gosch, Furr, & Sood, 2008) which proposes striking a balance between focusing on the client's wishes and needs and the therapist's provision of a structured intervention. Supervision for trainees or peer consultation for clinicians can be a particularly useful tool when undergoing such a process to provide support to the therapist trying to achieve the balance between the two.

Lastly, trainees and clinicians alike need to consider the challenges on a personal level of taking on the treatment and case management of such cases in the private sector. The work can be taxing emotionally and timewise. Even though one may derive satisfaction in helping clients through their struggles, one may wish to consider the importance and the need for self-care either in their caseload balance in terms of number of "challenging" cases they take on, or in seeking support via supervision or consultation to safeguard treatment adherence and ethical practice. Alternatively, if one wishes to focus on providing such services in the private sector, the clinician is strongly encouraged to consider building a professional team.

References

Beck, A. T., Rush, A. J., Shaw, B. F., & Emery, G. (1979). *Cognitive therapy of depression.* New York, NY: Guilford.

Chiang, K.-J., Tsai, J.-C., Liu, D., Lin, C.-H., Chiu, H.-L., & Chou, K.-R. (2017). Efficacy of cognitive-behavioral therapy in patients with bipolar disorder: A meta-analysis of randomized controlled trials. *PLoS One, 12*(5), e0176849. https://doi.org/10.1371/journal.pone.0176849

Geddes, J. R., & Miklowitz, D. J. (2013). Treatment of bipolar disorder. *Lancet, 381*(9878), 1672–1682. https://doi.org/10.1016/S0140-6736(13)60857-0

Johnson, S. L., & Miller, I. (1997). Negative life events and time to recovery from episodes of bipolar disorder. *Journal of Abnormal Psychology, 106*(3), 449–457. https://doi.org/10.1037//0021-843x.106.3.449

Kendall, P. C., & Frank, H. E. (2018). Implementing evidence-based treatment protocols: Flexibility within fidelity. *Clinical Psychology: Science and Practice, 25*(4), e12271. https://doi.org/10.1111/cpsp.12271

Kendall, P. C., Gosch, E., Furr, J. M., & Sood, E. (2008). Flexibility within fidelity. *Journal of the American Academy of Child & Adolescent Psychiatry, 47*(9), 987–993. https://doi.org/10.1097/CHI.0b013e31817eed2f

Miklowitz, D. J., Goldstein, M. J., Nuechterlein, K. H., Snyder, K. S., & Mintz, J. (1988). Family factors and the course of bipolar affective disorder. *Archives of General Psychiatry, 45,* 225–231. https://doi.org/10.1001/archpsyc.1988.01800270033004.

McMurrich, S. L., & Johnson, S. L. (2009). The role of depression, shame-proneness, and guilt-proneness in predicting criticism of relatives towards people with bipolar disorder. *Behavior Therapy, 40*(4), 315–324. https://doi.org/10.1016/j.beth.2008.09.003

Newman, C. F., Leahy, R. L., Beck, A. T., Reilly-Harrington, N. A., & Gyulai, L. (2001). *Bipolar disorder: A cognitive therapy approach.* Washington, DC: American Psychological Association.

Otto, M. W., Reilley-Harrington, N. A., & Sachs, G. S. (2003). Psychoeducation and cognitive-behavioral strategies in the management of bipolar disorder. *Journal of Affective Disorders, 73,* 171–181. https://doi.org/10.1016/S0165-0327(01)00460-8

Otto, M. W., Reilly-Harrington, N. A., Kogan, J. N., Henin, A., Knauz, R. O., & Sachs, G. S. (2009). *Managing bipolar disorder: A cognitive-behavioral approach (Therapist guide).* New York, NY: Oxford University Press.

Reilly-Harrington, N. A., Alloy, L. B., Fresco, D. M., & Whitehouse, W. G. (1999). Cognitive styles and life events interact to predict bipolar and unipolar symptomatology. *Journal of Abnormal Psychology, 108*(4), 567–578. https://doi.org/10.1037//0021-843x.108.4.567

Strauss, J. L., & Johnson, S. L. (2012). Role of treatment alliance in the clinical management of bipolar disorder: Stronger alliances prospectively predict fewer manic symptoms. *Psychiatry Research, 145*(2–3), 215–233. https://doi.org/10.1016/j.psychres.2006.01.007

Swartz, H. A., & Swanson, J. (2014). Psychotherapy for bipolar disorder in adults: A review of the evidence. *Focus, 12*(3), 251–266. https://doi.org/10.1176/appi.focus.12.3.251

Chapter 11
CBT and Psychodynamic Therapy: A Dialogue

Christos Charis and Georgia Panayiotou

Contents

CBT and psychodynamic therapists often look at each other suspiciously and harbor deep concerns about the effectiveness and validity of each others' approach. Indeed differences in both theory and practice are substantial, as can be observed by the chapters in this volume, written by experienced scholar/clinicians representing each view (and related approaches). Also, the two perspectives differ in the degree to which they rely on empirical data to support their effectiveness and their proposed mechanisms of disorder etiology and therapeutic change. This creates an additional difficulty in making comparisons. This brief discussion makes an attempt to summarize the main differences but also domains where the various approaches intersect, as shown by the chapters in this volume. We consider it a problem, for purposes of maintaining a fruitful dialogue among experienced clinicians across orientations, that the different schools do not recognize each other's value, in spite of the fact that several meta-analyses show effectiveness for each type of therapy and at least some meta-analytic evidence provides support for their equitable effects.

Unfortunately, in spite of its value for the current discussion, the meta-analytic evidence is not entirely conclusive when it comes to efficacy comparison. There is a large amount of data and randomized clinical trials reliably supporting the efficacy of CBT for a variety of disorders, and a number of meta-analyses show greater efficacy for CBT compared to psychodynamic treatment (PT), including with regards to depression (Grawe et al., 2004; Svartberg & Stiles, 1991; Tolin, 2010). However, these findings are somewhat skewed by the fact that fewer empirical studies exist to

C. Charis
Private Practice, Dillenburg, Germany

G. Panayiotou (✉)
Department of Psychology and Center of Applied Neuroscience, University of Cyprus, Nicosia, Cyprus
e-mail: georgiap@upcy.ap.cy

© Springer Nature Switzerland AG 2021
C. Charis, G. Panayiotou (eds.), *Depression Conceptualization and Treatment*,
https://doi.org/10.1007/978-3-030-68932-2_11

test psychodynamically oriented therapy, which is often not manualized or time-limited, and few well-conducted comparative studies exist. Other meta-analytic studies tend to find comparable effects for CBT and structured short-term psychodynamic psychotherapy (STPP; e.g., Leichsenring, 2001) as well as other therapies (Shedler, 2010). With regard to P, PT several recent studies support that it is an effective treatment (Jacobsen et al., 2007; Keller, 2013). As Professor Benecke writes, there is hardly any doubt about the effectiveness of the methods (Benecke, 2016; Wampold & Imel, 2015). Findings, however, should still be received with some caution as both CBT and STPP are not always applied in practice with the same structured, manualized manner included in the efficacy studies. More research is clearly needed to offer more conclusive data. In the absence of such empirical support, let us focus on some descriptive aspects to help us compare and contrast these approaches. The reader can gain understanding of the richness of each individual approach by looking at the chapters of this volume.

Psychodynamic teaching is based on the following concepts: *the unconscious, the conflicts* derived from it and from *drive and motivation theory, affects* and their *defense processes, transference* and *countertransference*, as well as formative relationship experiences (*representations*).

The "unconscious" goes back to Freud (1900). Freud distinguishes three forms of consciousness: the unconscious, the preconscious, and the conscious ("The Topical Model"; 1923). With "preconscious" mental processes are meant, which easily enter consciousness when focusing attention on these preconscious contents. According to Freud, the unconscious is a psychological instance whose function is to keep psychodynamically acting impulses, ideas, feelings, and desires away from consciousness because they are conflictual, thus relieving the person of neurotic stress. ("Neurotically relieved" means that the individual is relieved but at the price that neurotic symptoms develop.) It is a dynamic term. Another construct that is closely linked to the unconscious is the defense mechanisms that Anna Freud (1936) defined in detail. The defense switches on "automatically" and aims to regulate painful feelings, impulses, affects, etc., by keeping these contents unconscious. Although it has an ego function with protective and coping tasks, it is ultimately dysfunctional in the context of neurotic conflicts (Mentzos, 1984. Hoffmann, Hochapfel, Eckhardt-Henn, & Heuft, 2004). The question of what makes people mentally ill, in this case depressed, is answered today by psychodynamic theory as follows:

1. Man or woman has basic needs. If these needs are not met in the first years of life, the person concerned becomes susceptible to mental illness. The disappointment of these needs leads to the development of neurotic conflicts, which become pathogenic in later life.
2. The individual becomes ill due to structural deficits that arise in the course of the individual's psychological development and manifest themselves in threshold situations in life.
3. Trauma.

The following needs are relevant for the manifestation of depression: First is need for attachment—search for love and attachment in the relationship with others. For example, the mother is very hardened due to her own biographical experiences and has not learned to love. The child cannot recognize: "I am lovable, but my mother cannot love." It thinks, "I'm not lovable myself." It experiences itself helpless and learns to resign itself quickly (e.g., Bowlby, 1969). The second is the need for regulation of the own self-esteem (Kohut, 1979). The third is need for autonomy and individuation which is an equally central theme (Mahler, Pine, & Bergman, 1978). In the separation phase (second year of life), in which the child's first major development of autonomy takes place, the second disturbance of depressive vulnerability lies (Blatt & Homann, 1992). During this period, the child begins to develop a sense of self-worth and identity. Disorders here can lead to the formation of anger and resentment in interpersonal relationships and to a devalued self-image, which is associated with pronounced feelings of shame, guilt, and a feeling of not being enough. The children remain bound to the primary persons but in an insecure-ambivalent or insecure-avoiding way. In a third focus of disturbance in the oedipal period of the fifth and sixth years, we encounter the consolidation of the superego. Here, the depressively vulnerable children have an increased tendency to feel guilt and shame and a tendency to self-criticism and feelings of failure. This is probably also where the characterological paths finally separate: whether the children tend toward the dependent- and object-related type and regressively avoid the Oedipus conflict or whether they develop in the self-critical and autonomous direction and expand their progressive defenses. The specific way in which the depressives have failed to cope with the Oedipal situation lies in their avoidance and evasion. They avoid Oedipal confrontation with the respective same-sex parent. This is how self-doubt as a man or woman comes about this is how self-doubt as a man or woman comes about, because their is a lack of identification with the same-sex parent, and tendency to feelings of guilt and depression, because a man who is Oedipally fixated feels like a failure and therefore cannot compete because he is prone to feelings of guilt (Will, Grabenstedt, Völkl, & Banck, 2008. Busch, Rudden, & Shapiro, 2016). A large part of these needs or conflicts is also presented in Dr. Charis' Chap. 6 on the basis of the problems analyzed there ("anaclitic" (fears of abandonment; dependency) versus "intIn a thirdrojective" (hash self-criticism; perfectionism)). Neurotic conflicts are mobilized by triggering situations, whereby their pathogenic effect comes into play and the person concerned becomes depressed. For psychodynamic therapy it is important to record the triggering moments, because these provide information about the psychodynamic background of the disorder on which the therapy is based. For example, the fact that a patient becomes depressed after the death of his mother diagnostically indicates a conflict with his inner image of his mother, which is updated by the death of the real mother. In this case, the conflict could be, "I did not get enough love from my mother, but until now I had the unconscious hope that one day I would experience enough love. But now that my mother has died, my last hope is also disappointed!" As a result of the actualization of the conflict at hand, the conflict is formed during a certain phase of psychological development in the first 6 years of life, the intensity of the affect becomes stronger (in the case of grief and other depressive symptoms), and the defense and depressive symptoms are formed as a solution to the conflict. Furthermore, from a psychodynamic point of view, the structure of the personality plays an important role in the manifestation of depression, whereby conflict pathology and structural pathology are not mutually exclusive. What is "structure of personality"? This refers to basic psychological functions of the ego, the degree of maturity of which determines the personality of a person. Basic qualities of mental functioning (so-called structural level) are recorded. An important example of this is the structural concept of mentalization. At this point I would like to refer to Chap. 3 by Dr. Bilger in this book. The working group of the OPD (Arbeitskreis, 2006) comprises structural abilities in four areas, whereby these abilities have an internal and external reference: ability to perceive oneself and the important others, to control (i.e., to regulate impulses, affects, self-esteem in the case of offenses; to regulate relationships by taking one's own interests and those of the others into account appropriately), to communicate (emotional communication: developing and experiencing one's own affects, fantasies; allowing and expressing feelings toward the others; empathy), and to bond (being bound to inner and outer objects). For example, if people cannot be helped because they are not bound, this can increase their depression.

Other important concepts of psychodynamic theory are transference and representations. Representations (unconscious inner psychic relationship patterns) are formed as a result of relationship experiences mainly in childhood. Thus self-representations and representations of significant others, so-called object representations, develop. They represent condensations of early affective experiences, but they are not always the reflection of past real experiences. They can be understood as a kind of unconscious templates that are activated by interactions in everyday life. The representations have a strong influence on the way the person experiences the world, and as a result they shape their relationship behavior, which can be dysfunctional. Luborsky and Chrits-Christoph (1998) speak of "core conflictual relationship themes," meaning unconscious beliefs that are expressed in everyday situations. A baby, for example, who experiences with his depressed mother that his mother is not really present for the child, first tries to make his needs clear. In the course of time and if his mother's response is still lacking, the baby begins to look away and avoid eye contact. It turns more and more to a self-comforting behavior. Probably such people have the expectation that they will not get an answer to their activities and that they will not get any help in regulating their own affects and arousals. This confirms the findings of René Spitz (Spitz & Wolf, 1946), who studied babies in American children's homes in the 1940s who had experienced comparable states of loneliness and had developed early childhood anaclitic depression. Such a child may become convinced that it is unable to reach the object and is therefore thrown back on itself. He may internalize this as a disinterest in the object, and he may feel at the mercy of his own affects, emotions, fantasies, and fears and may gain the attitude that he has to cope with himself, even if he is not able to do so at all. In later stages of development, it may internalize disappointment and rejection as an essential part of object relationships (object representations), and it may link the question of why the mother rejects it with guilt attributes and say to itself:

"I am to blame for the reasons that I am doing so badly" (self-representation). Examples of this can be found in Chap. 6 by Dr. Charis. The representative offices form the basis for the so-called transfer. It is the tendency to revive earlier relationship patterns out of the need to satisfy unfulfilled infantile desires and longings, to resolve unresolved conflicts, or to prevent ascending fears. According to Freud, transmission is a misunderstanding of the present in terms of the past (Freud, 1912). The transference of depressive people is explained in more detail in Chap. 5 by Professor Busch. Behavioral therapy also understands representations as the precipitation of early experiences that strongly determine behavior.

Psychodynamic therapy (PT) has empathy and a strong therapeutic alliance as an important prerequisite for successful treatment. It enables the patient to engage with the experiences underlying his pathogenic beliefs with the associated negative affective content and thus gain emotional insight. These new experiences are internalized by the patient according to psychodynamic ideas. New representations arise. The analytic functions of the therapist are internalized, for example, the way in which he works out connections and commonalities, how he deals with affects, etc. (Thomä & Kächele, 2006). A depressive patient recently told me, "When I recently wrote an e-mail to the administration of my employer and they did not answer me, I thought, 'What would my therapist say or do now?' So I decided to call them instead of giving up like I usually do." An important questionnaire for recording the therapeutic alliance is the Working Alliance Inventory by Horvath and Greenberg (1989). The influence of the therapeutic alliance on the success of treatment is considered an important moderating factor for success. A direct curative effect is not assumed (Kazdin, 2009). It is very important that the therapist behaves differently than the patient's unconscious relationship expectations that have arisen from early experiences suggest.

In addition, countertransference is of central importance in psychodynamic therapy. Countertransference is understood to be the therapist's inner psychological reactions, for example, emotions, fantasies, etc., due to the patient's interactive influence on the therapist. It is important as a therapist to become aware of these mostly unconscious inner reactions, because they become like a key to the inner world of the patient. An example of this is the countertransference in Chap. 6 by Dr. Charis "Therapy." The core of psychodynamic work is the transmission of emotional insight. Emotional insight serves to help the patient to consciously experience emotionally the desires and affects (guilt, fear, anger, grief, etc.) that have been warded off until then and to become aware of the until then unconscious attachments in old relationship patterns. A mere remembering without the activation of affects in the here and now of the treatment situation is not healing (Freud, 1912). As a result of emotional insight, infantile unconscious aspects of the individual become conscious and thus lose their unconscious power over their experience and actions. The classical means of conveying emotional insight is the work of interpretation. It is the formulation of an assumption about an unconscious context of meaning. The therapist first tries to grasp and formulate the patient's current main problem and then to understand his unconscious background so that he can establish a causal connection. For this purpose the patient needs a space to unfold his unconscious pathogenic patterns. After this patient work, the therapist tries to gently guide the patient toward the latter's unconscious and painful affects. If this succeeds, new self and object representations are created, which contribute to the patient's better quality of life. Here is an example with a depressive patient from the therapeutic everyday life. After the end of the first 12 therapy sessions, Mr. S initially shows himself willing to submit another application to the health insurance company so that the costs for the therapy still to be carried out can be covered. But by reflecting on himself, he realizes that he himself does not really want to prolong the therapy because he thought that the most important issues had been discussed and that he was feeling better. However, the therapist has the hypothesis that the depressed patient does not want to continue the therapy because he fears something, e.g., being disappointed. Against this background, the therapist decides on the following interpretation: Mr. S does not want to prolong the therapy because he probably has the concern that he will get more involved with the therapist and could be disappointed. This interpretation puts Mr. S in a reflective mood. He then explains to the therapist that he is afraid he might disappoint the therapist because he is not good enough. Therefore he does not want to stay in therapy any longer. Mr. S then asks for a week to think about it. At the next session, he says that he himself had also come to the conclusion that there was actually a lot to discuss, so he wanted to stay in therapy.

Let us now turn to the fundamental concepts on which cognitive behavioral therapy (CBT) approaches lie. Although historically evolving out of the psychoanalytic tradition, early founders of this approach, like Beck, Ellis, Bandura, and others, placed more emphasis of the therapeutic process in the "here and now," that is, in the current determinants and maintenance factors of behavior, as compared to its developmental roots. Therapy comes about when the contingencies and mechanisms that maintain current symptoms and maladaptive behavioral patterns are modified to encourage more adaptive responses. The therapy is an active, solution-focused process, where the therapist acts as a coach, teacher, and role model but where the client is an active agent, engaging in exercises, planned activities, and experiments that will enhance discovery and generalize therapeutic gains outside the therapy session. Based on a general commitment to scientific validation, the CBT therapist will collaborate with the psychiatrist and other mental health professionals where the science indicates that such a collaboration will enhance outcome, e.g., where pharmacotherapy or family therapy has been shown to improve therapy effectiveness. Examples of treatment approaches for depression in both private practice, hospital setting and the health sector, are presented by several of the authors of Chaps. 4, 10, and 9 in this volume, including Jackson et al., Karayianni, and Zacharia and Karekla.

In CBT, strong emphasis is placed on current thoughts, emotions, and behaviors, the inter-relationship among them, and what triggers and maintains them. Also, CBT, as most contemporary therapies, recognizes the fact that humans are biopsychosocial animals and that psychopathology also has a biological side, as clearly demonstrated in Chap. 1 by Chatzittofis in this volume, and takes into consideration contemporary findings from neuroscience, experimental psychology, and genetics to inform understanding of the reasons why a particular client is vulnerable to a particular cluster of symptoms, as in the case of depression. Similarly, individuals live in social contexts, which influence and shape their perceptions and schemas and selectively reinforce behaviors. The social context of depression is nicely addressed in Chap. 2 by Orphanidou and Kadianaki.

Having said this, a comprehensive case formulation based on CBT approaches does not remain at the level of describing current maintenance patterns for behavior. Predisposing factors, like family history, traumatic events, and temperamental characteristics, for example, trait neuroticism, are assessed and evaluated for their contribution to the current clinical presentation. Precipitants of the current clinical episode and triggers of repeated episodes, whether environmental, interpersonal, or internal (i.e., specific thoughts or experiences), are identified and recorded. Also, the strengths and weaknesses that the client brings to therapy are considered as they may impact the outcome. Based on a science-informed model of generating and supporting or refuting hypotheses about the pathogenic mechanisms, CBT proponents stress this approach's links to empiricism and typically rely heavily on protocols that have been shown reliably to be effective on the basis of randomized clinical trials. However, given large individual differences in response, adapting and adjusting the implementation of protocols to the circumstances of individual clients is encouraged, as seen in the case study by Karayianni in this volume.

Starting with the fundamental difference between PT and CBT, it is apparent that they have a different approach to their disease models and the therapy strategies used. While PT considers the therapeutic relationship as a main vehicle of change, CBT and behavior therapy focus on learning principles and experiences. Patients learn particular patterns of behavior through social learning and modeling of important figures (Bandura & Walters, 1963) and through operant and classical reinforcement principles (Pavlov, 1897; Skinner, 1938; Watson, 1924). Through such principles, they don't only learn overt behaviors but also more covert behaviors such as stereotypic/irrational thoughts and assumptions (Beck, 1967; Ellis, 1957) and emotional responses such as phobic reactions (Wolpe, 1969). The therapist, then, is called to act as a role model and coach and facilitate the patient to identify the contingencies that maintain dysfunctional behaviors, thoughts, and emotional responses and collaboratively shape the contingencies to create new, corrective learning experiences. Chapters 8, 9, and 4 by Panayiotou, Zacharia and Karekla, and Björgvinsson et al. clearly delineate the theoretical underpinnings and therapeutic methods that characterize behavior and cognitive aspects of therapy as well as third wave approaches. However, the value of the therapeutic relationship is not any smaller in CBT. Like PT, CBT "utilizes" the therapist as a vehicle of change. The therapist acts as a role model, demonstrating adaptive behaviors and responses both as part of role plays and psychoeducation and as part of the interpersonal interactions with the client. The therapist, using the significance of the relationship with the patient, monitors reinforcement contingencies, providing praise and differential reinforcement for patient behaviors.

More elements exist where these approaches intersect, in spite of their fundamental differences. As shown by a large body of both classical and more recent psychotherapy research, in addition to the specific curative elements of each psychotherapeutic approach, all psychotherapies share common characteristics or elements that explain a substantial amount of variance in the observed improvement. These include the fact that the problem of the patient receives meaning through the formulation of the reported problems, the fact that there is normalization of one's experience, benefit from empathy and support offered by the therapist, and gaining hope about solving one's difficulties, among others.

Turning to the central similarities between PT and CBT, we can identify common elements in conceptualization and active treatment components, albeit with different emphasis and terminology. In terms of the interpersonal elements of psychotherapy, any seasoned therapist, irrespective of their theoretical approach, will stress the value of a trusting therapeutic relationship, as discussed above in the context of PT. The work alliance is regarded as a necessary prerequisite for the patient to engage in the treatment (Kanfer, Reinecker, & Schmelzer, 2000) in both approaches.

Another determinant of success is that (as discussed in Chap. 6 by Charis on psychodynamic therapy) therapist and patient need to arrive to a shared understanding of the problem (insight). In CBT terms, this will lead to a common agenda between therapist and patient, while in more psychodynamic terms, the client will gain insight into the sources of their difficulties. There will be little progress if the client does not "buy into" the conceptualization and the rationale for the proposed interventions. Unless the client is convinced that the therapist hears and empathizes with their pain, and that the proposed interventions, through the jointly understood mechanism of change, will ultimately lead to a reduction in pain, the client will have difficulty engaging with the therapy. He or she may find themselves diverging to other topics of discussion beyond the agenda (or the central topic), terminating early, or participating without making progress. Such an attitude in psychodynamic terms might constitute resistance rooted in similar reasons: The client doesn't feel heard, acknowledged, or valued and has reasons (or reinforcement contingencies as would be called in behavioral terms) to maintain one's current behavior. In other words, to the client, the costs of losing the current pattern of behaviors ultimately appears to outweigh the benefit of adopting new, adaptive ways of coping. This cost entails the fear of change and of meeting new challenges that is an inevitable obstacle in all therapy. We often tell our trainees that in order for clients to feel comfortable letting go of old, well-practiced but maladaptive ways of coping, they need to learn, practice, and feel sure about the new ways they are told about in therapy. Expecting them to drop their old ways before having over-learned and accepted new approaches as suitable for them, and trusting that their therapist is acting on their best interest, is like pulling the carpet from under their feet! Thus, both CBT traditions and psychodynamic therapy rest on the necessary element of therapeutic trust and a common understanding achieved between client and therapist. In terms of differences in this domain, indeed the therapeutic relationship plays a stronger therapeutic role in PT, through transference, an element less important in CBT. However, it should be noted that experienced CBT therapists closely observe the interpersonal process of therapy, and note patterns of interactions that likely reflect similar maladaptive behaviors in the outside world, using them as examples to train in new skills and identify negative automatic thoughts.

Another common element pertains to the formulation of the problem itself, as understood by therapist and client. As noted above, irrespective of the theoretical approach, an understanding of the mechanisms that connect different presenting problems and provide a glimpse of how these problems might change instills hope and provides meaning. Using a case formulation, based primarily on the clinical interview and secondarily on test results and low-level clinical inference (Eells, 1997), may be a common element for the psychotherapies discussed in this volume. Almost inevitably, these formulations, irrespective of the theory, will contain elements about the way the client sees/interprets themselves, the world, and their future (i.e., automatic thoughts, core beliefs, introjected views of the self, unconscious representations/schemas), many of which were based on past experiences and relationships. Although PT may invest a much greater percentage of time exploring the historical sources of these cognitions and stereotypes, CBT, though focusing more on the present and future, acknowledges the role of the past in formulating current thinking and behavior. Indeed, as indicated in Chap. 8 by Panayiotou, CBT may focus on historical examples as evidence in order to help the client dispute maladaptive core beliefs. Thus, in spite of the emphasis of CBT approaches on the present, both CBT and psychodynamic approaches often take a developmental perspective in their case formulations, identifying the learning sources of strongly held beliefs and stereotypes in the past.

Some of the core therapeutic techniques used by the approaches described in this book may rest on similar underlying psychological mechanisms, in spite of being described differently by each approach. A central approach to CBT, and especially behavior therapy, involves exposure, used primarily to treat anxiety problems, OCD, and PTSD (but also eating disorders and substance use). Exposure, systematic desensitization (Wolpe & Wolpe, 1988), or progressive application of new skills in domains that were previously avoided is also central to behavioral activation, as discussed by Panayiotou. Although a cornerstone of CBT, known to be a potent active component of therapeutic change, exposure-like components are found in many non-CBT therapies such as paradoxical intention, emotionally focused therapy, self-psychology, and interpersonal psychotherapy. Furthermore, having thoughts, feelings, fantasies, and other mental material that was previously unconscious (because it was intolerable) become part of awareness (and thus become to some degree tolerable) is a central mechanism of psychodynamic therapies. It is considered to lead to catharsis, ridding the person of intrapsychic pain. In spite of the differences in concepts, presumed mechanisms and terminologies, being consciously "exposed" to this mental content and to painful realities, are perhaps not dissimilar to exposure therapy, as practiced, for example, in PTSD and OCD. Through learning that one can tolerate and cope with what was previously considered as intolerable, integrating it with one's current self-concept, and dismissing one's conscious or unconscious predictions that this contact would be catastrophic (Craske, Treanor, Conway, Zbozinek, & Vervliet, 2014) seems to be another common element that brings on substantial therapeutic strides, across therapeutic traditions.

Inevitably, most patients will seek therapy because of difficult emotions, whether these involve anger, anxiety, depression, or flat and inappropriate affect, leading to interpersonal ineffectiveness. Another similarity then between both (and all) psychotherapeutic approaches is the focus on emotions. Difficulties in emotion regulation and emotion processing are paramount in psychopathology, and all of human suffering. Ineffective attempts to regulate unwanted emotions, which may be called coping in CBT and defense mechanisms in PT, are necessarily the target of therapy, irrespective of perspective, and a fundamental hypothesized mechanism of the presenting problems. Emotion regulation through avoidance (e.g., denial, substance use), rumination, or blaming can lead to maintenance of problems. Therapy will help in the identification of emotions and their triggers of these maladaptive ways of regulating them and help substitute them with more adaptive ways. In PT terms, this understanding will be called insight. In CBT, this knowledge comes about from the process of collaborative discovery. Although the mechanism through which this change is achieved may be somewhat different, the goal and the result are quite similar across perspectives (Westen, 1994). Patients, either through the corrective experiences offered by the therapeutic relationship, or the new learning experiences jointly decided through homework and other exercises, acquire the ability to tolerate affect that was previously intolerable and to respond to affect-laden situations in more flexible ways, consistent with the demands of the context but also with one's values and life goals. Recent developments in third wave approaches like acceptance and commitment therapy (see Chap. 9 by Zacharia and Karekla) specifically encourage emotional awareness through mindfulness and acceptance, and attempt to decrease avoidance, which is believed to play a defensive role against unwanted experiences— such terminology is not far divergent from traditional PT conceptualizations.

Many other similarities can be identified: Experienced and respectful practitioners can see similar processes unfolding in the process of therapy that ultimately lead to improvement. These reflect common elements but also distinct curative components that may have different names and follow different procedures but ultimately help to address dysfunctions in similar underlying processes and mechanisms. Developments in neuroscience, genetics, and biology may help us to describe more specifically in the future the specific changes in brain circuits and psychological systems that our therapeutic efforts help to modify in ways that produce clinically significant change. In the meantime, respectful dialogues between practitioners across perspectives can enrich our understanding of our own work and help us see our patients as the complex and interesting beings that they are.

References

Arbeitskreis (2006). *Operationalisierte Psychodynamische Diagnostik OPD-2. Das Manual für Diagnostik und Therapieplanung*. Bern.
Bandura, A., & Walters, R. H. (1963). *Social learning and personality development*. New York, NY: Holt, Rinehart, & Winston.

Beck, A. T. (1967). *Depression: Causes and treatment*. Philadelphia, PA: University of Pennsylvania Press.

Benecke, C. (2016). *Psychodynamische Therapien und Verhaltenstherapie im Vergleich*. Göttingen: Vandenhoeck & Ruprecht.

Blatt, S. J., & Homann, E. (1992). Parent-child interaction in the etiology of dependent and self-critical depression. *Clinical psychology review, 12*(1), 47–91.

Bowlby, J. (1969). *Bindung. Eine Analyse der Mutter-Kind-Beziehung*. München: Kindler.

Busch, F. N., Rudden, M., & Shapiro, T. (2016). *Psychodynamic treatment of depression*. Washington, DC: American Psychiatric Pub.

Craske, M. G., Treanor, M., Conway, C. C., Zbozinek, T., & Vervliet, B. (2014). Maximizing exposure therapy: An inhibitory learning approach. *Behaviour Research and Therapy, 58*, 10–23.

Ellis, A. (1957). Rational psychotherapy and individual psychology. *Journal of Individual Psychology, 13*, 38–44.

Eells, T. D. (1997). Psychotherapy case formulation: History and current status. In T. D. Eells (Ed.), Handbook of psychotherapy case formulation (p. 1–25). Guilford Press.

Freud, A. (1936). *Das Ich und die Abwehrmechanismen*. München: Kindler.

Freud, S. (1900). *Die Traumdeutung. GW II/III*. London: Imago.

Freud, S. (1912). *Zur Dynamik der Übertragung. GW VIII* (pp. 157–168). London: Imago.

Freud, S. (1923). *das Ich und das Es. GW XIII* (pp. 237–289). London: Imago.

Grawe, K. (2004). Psychological therapy. Hogrefe Publishing.

Hoffmann, S. O., Hochapfel, G., Eckhardt-Henn, A., & Heuft, G. (2004). *Neurotische Störungen und Psychosomatische Medizin: Mit einer Einführung in Psychosomatik und Psychotherapie*. Stuttgart: Schattauer.

Horvath, A. O., & Greenberg, L. S. (1989). Development and validation of the working alliance inventory. *Journal of Counseling Psychology, 36*, 223–233.

Jacobsen, T., Rudolf, G., Brockmann, J., Eckert, J., Huber, D., Klug, G., … Leichsenring, F. (2007). Ergebnisse analytischer Psychotherapien bei spezifischen psychischen Störungen. Verbesserungen in der Symptomatik und in den interpersonellen Beziehungen. *Zeitschrift für Psychosomatische Medin und Psychotherapie, 53*, 87–110.

Kanfer, F. H., Reinecker, H., & Schmelzer, D. (2000). *Selbstmanagement-Therapie-ein Lehrbuch für die Praxis*. Berlin: Springer.

Kazdin, A. E. (2009). Understanding ho wand why psychotherapy leads to change. *Psychotherapy Research, 19*, 418–428.

Keller, W. (2013). Symptomatik und strukturelle Veränderungen bei chronisch depressiven Patienten. Teilergebnis der Praxisstudie analytische Langzeittherapie (PAL-Studie). In M. Leuzinger-Bohleber, U. Bahrke, & A. Negele (Eds.), *Chronische Depression: Verstehen – Behandeln – Erforschen*. Göttingen: Vandenhoeck & Ruprecht.

Kohut, H. (1979). *Die Heilung des Selbst*. Frankfurt am Main: Suhrkamp.

Luborsky, L., & Chrits-Christoph, P. (1998). *Understanding transference. The core conflictual relationship theme method* (2nd ed.). New York, NY: Basic Books.

Leichsenring, F. (2001). Comparative effects of short-term psychodynamic psychotherapy and cognitive-behavioral therapy in depression: a meta-analytic approach. *Clinical psychology review*, Elsevier.

Mahler, M. S., Pine, F., & Bergman, A. (1978). *Die psychische Geburt des Menschen*. Frankfurt am Main: Fischer.

Mentzos, S. (1984). *Neurotische Konfliktverarbeitung*. Frankfurt am Main: Fischer.

Pavlov, I. P. (1897/1902). *The work of the digestive glands*. London: Griffin.

Shedler, J. (2010). The efficacy of psychodynamic psychotherapy. *American psychologist, 65*(2), 98.

Skinner, B. F. (1938). *The behavior of organisms. An experimental analysis*. New York, NY: Appleton-Century-Croft.

Spitz, R.A., Wolf K.M. (1946) Anaclitic depression: An inquiry into the genesis of psychiatric conditions in early childhood, II. Volume 2, 313–342.

Svartberg, M., & Stiles, T. C. (1991). Comparative effects of short-term psychodynamic psycho-therapy: a meta-analysis. *Journal of consulting and clinical psychology, 59*(5), 704.

Thomä, H., & Kächele, H. (2006). *Lehrbuch der psychoanalytischen Therapie. Band I.* Berlin: Springer.

Tolin, D. F. (2010). Is cognitive–behavioral therapy more effective than other therapies?: A meta-analytic review. *Clinical psychology review, 30*(6), 710–720.

Wampold, B. E., & Imel, Z. E. (2015). *The great psychotherapy debate. The evidence for what makes psychotherapy works* (2nd ed.). New York, NY: Routledge.

Watson, J. B. (1924). *Behaviorism.* New York, NY: People's Institute Publishing Company.

Will, H., Grabenstedt, Y., Völkl, G., & Banck, G. (2008). *Depression. Psychodynamik und Therapie. 3 überarbeitete und erweiterte Auflage.* Stuttgart: W. Kohlhammer.

Wolpe, J. (1969). Basic principles and practices of behavior therapy of neuroses. *American Journal of Psychiatry, 125*(9), 1242–1247.

Wolpe, J., & Wolpe, D. (1988). Life without fear. New Harbinger Publications.

Westen, D. (1994). Implications of cognitive science for psychotherapy: Promises and limitations.

Index

A
Acceptance and commitment therapy (ACT), 43, 44
  acceptance, internal experiences, 127
  aims, 123
  assessment of progress, 141, 142
  for cancer patients, 125
  case of KC, 127
  and CBT, 123
  cognitive fusion, 124
  experiential avoidance, 124, 132 (*see also* Experiential avoidance)
  external barriers/obstacles, 138
  functional behavioral analysis, 127
  hypothetical mechanism, 136
  precipitating factors, 130, 131
  presenting problems
    behavior, 129
    emotions/physical sensations, 129
    thoughts and memories, 128
  processes, 127
  in psychological and physical health problems, 126
  psychological flexibility, 123, 131
  termination and relapse prevention, 141
  theory-driven behavioral approach, 123
  treatment plan, 138
  values-consistent life, 125
Adrenocorticotropic hormone (ACTH), 4, 5
Aggression, 56, 57, 59
Alcohol abuse, 11
Alprazolam, 10
Anger, 55, 61, 77
Anger management skills, 158
Anxiety, 32, 35

Assertiveness skills, 159
Attachment theory, 57
Attention bias modification therapy (ABMT), 117
Attention biases, 110
Autoaggressive symptoms, 35

B
Behavioral activation (BA), 42, 43, 113, 114
Behavioral Health Partial Hospital Program (BHP)
  BA, 42
  CBT, 42
  clinical data collection, 47
  clinical information, 45
  clinical team, 40
  clinical work, 48
  diagnosis, 48
  McLean Hospital, 40
  multiple comorbidities, 44
  panic attack, 45
  PHP setting, 38, 42
  research, 40, 48
  third-wave approaches, 43
  training program, 49
Behavioral withdrawal, 112
Behaviour therapy, 75
Biases, 109, 117
Biomarkers, 4, 18
Biopsychosocial model, 19
Bipolar disorder, 21, 149
  and cannabis use, 152, 153, 161, 162
  mental health issues, 151
Bipolar-focused treatments, 150